NATIONAL DEFENSE RESEARCH INSTITUTE

T0127952

Care Transitions to and from the National Intrepid Center of Excellence (NICoE) for Service Members with Traumatic Brain Injury

Lynsay Ayer, Coreen Farris, Carrie M. Farmer, Lily Geyer, Dionne Barnes-Proby, Gery W. Ryan, Lauren Skrabala, Deborah M. Scharf

Prepared for the Office of the Secretary of Defense
Approved for public release; distribution unlimited

For more information on this publication, visit www.rand.org/t/RR653

Library of Congress Cataloging-in-Publication Data is available for this publication.
ISBN: 978-0-8330-8888-8

Published by the RAND Corporation, Santa Monica, Calif.

© Copyright 2015 RAND Corporation

RAND® is a registered trademark.

Support RAND
Make a tax-deductible charitable contribution at
www.rand.org/giving/contribute

www.rand.org

Preface

Since 2001, more than 2 million U.S. service members have deployed in support of Operation Enduring Freedom and Operation Iraqi Freedom. In these conflicts, improvised explosive devices (IEDs) have been one of the leading causes of death and injury among U.S. troops. Those who survive an IED blast or other injuries related to combat exposure, training accidents, or motor vehicle accidents may be left with a traumatic brain injury (TBI) and attendant or co-occurring psychological symptoms. In response to the need for specialized services for these populations, the U.S. Department of Defense (DoD) established the National Intrepid Center of Excellence (NICoE) in Bethesda, Maryland, in 2010.

The NICoE's mission is to provide interdisciplinary diagnostic evaluations and treatment planning for comorbid TBI and psychological health conditions with the goal of supporting service members' ability to continue active-duty service, or successfully transition to civilian life. Service members from across the country travel to the NICoE to receive specialized assessments and individualized treatment planning and then return to their home stations, where local providers are expected to implement the NICoE treatment plans.

Because service members spend only four weeks at the NICoE and continue their treatment at their home stations, the NICoE's success in fulfilling its mission is impacted by its relationships with home station providers, patients, and their families. The RAND Corporation was asked to evaluate these relationships and provide recommendations for strengthening the NICoE's efforts to communicate with these groups to improve attending to patients' TBI care. Through surveys, site visits, and interviews with NICoE staff, home station providers, service members who have received care at the NICoE, and the families of these patients, RAND's evaluation examined the interactions between the NICoE and the providers responsible for referring patients to the NICoE and implementing treatment plans. The evaluation identified a range of factors influencing providers' decisions to refer patients to the NICoE, the process by which the NICoE's recommendations are communicated to home station providers, and the ease with which the recommendations are implemented after a patient's stay at the NICoE has concluded. This report includes a series of recommendations for the NICoE as it seeks to better meet the needs of the population it serves, and as NICoE satellite facilities open across the country.

This report will be of interest to decisionmakers in the U.S. Department of Defense who are involved in planning and allocating funding for services and programs designed to meet these needs of service members with TBI and psychological health conditions, as well as providers who work with this military population. The findings should also be useful to NICoE decisionmakers responsible for program planning and quality improvement of NICoE processes and for home station providers interested in understanding more about the NICoE's roles and responsibilities.

This research was sponsored by the Defense Centers of Excellence for Psychological Health and Traumatic Brain Injury (DCoE) and conducted within the Forces and Resources Policy Center of the RAND National Defense Research Institute, a federally funded research and development center sponsored by the Office of the Secretary of Defense, the Joint Staff, the Unified Combatant Commands, the Navy, the Marine Corps, the defense agencies, and the defense Intelligence Community. For more information on the RAND Forces and Resources Policy Center, see http://www.rand.org/nsrd/ndri/centers/frp.html or contact the director (contact information is provided on the web page).

Contents

Figures

Tables

Summary

Between 2001 and 2011, 2.2 million U.S. service members were deployed in support of Operation Enduring Freedom (OEF) and Operation Iraqi Freedom (OIF). These conflicts have resulted in long, frequent deployments for many of these service members, as well as historically high levels of participation by reserve forces. Although most service members cope well with deployment-related stresses, the wartime risks of the past decade have led to significant rates of physical injuries and psychological health problems.

Improvised explosive devices (IEDs), used extensively against U.S. forces in OEF and OIF, have been one of the leading causes of death and injury. Traumatic brain injury (TBI)—a frequent consequence of these IED blasts—has been called the signature injury of these conflicts. TBIs are not exclusively a combat injury, however. They can also result from training accidents, motor vehicle accidents, and other traumas. Depending on the severity, a TBI can include a loss or decrease of consciousness and can result in memory problems, confusion or disorientation, or neurological deficits (such as weakness, a loss of balance, and sensory changes).

Compared to service members who have never experienced a TBI, those who have are more likely to develop a psychiatric disorder, such as posttraumatic stress disorder (PTSD) or depression. Although recovery can occur without formal care, service members benefit from formal diagnostics, assessment, and treatment to help them to regain their original capabilities and return to full duty. For those for whom a full recovery and return to duty is not feasible, these same services can help them to adjust to their new baseline and effectively transition out of the service.

While the military health care system has adjusted proactively to meet the unique needs of service members recovering from physical and psychological injuries, not all patients can be optimally served by the standard infrastructure of local military treatment facilities. A small proportion of these patients may benefit from specialty services designed to treat comorbid TBI and psychological health conditions.

In response to this need for specialty services, the U.S. Department of Defense (DoD) opened the National Intrepid Center of Excellence (NICoE) in Bethesda, Maryland, in 2010. The NICoE provides interdisciplinary diagnostic evaluations, short-term treatment, and treatment planning for comorbid TBI and psychological health conditions with the goal of mitigating barriers some service members face in seeking treatment and supporting service members' ability to return to full service. Service members from across the country travel to the NICoE for a four-week stay, where they receive specialized assessments and individualized treatment plans. They then return to their home bases, with the expectation that local providers will implement these treatment plans. The NICoE facility accepts five new patients per week, for a total of 20 patients per month. At the time of this evaluation, approximately 400 service members had received services at the NICoE.

NICoE administrators and staff view comprehensive assessment, development of customized treatment plans, and education of the patient and family members as their primary clinical aims. The facility supports state-of-the-art diagnostic testing. In addition, the NICoE provides traditional and alternative treatments such as group counseling, psychoeducation, yoga, Tai Chi, and service dog training. Given the short stay, these treatments are also considered assessments. That is, patients engage in the treatment modality during their stay in order to assess whether continued engagement with a given treatment approach would be beneficial and should be added to their long-term treatment plan.

Because service members spend only four weeks at the NICoE and continue their treatment at their home stations, the NICoE's success in addressing the needs of service members and their families is impacted to a great degree by its relationships with home station providers, patients, and their families.

Evaluation Approach

The RAND Corporation was asked to evaluate the complex communication and relationships between the NICoE, home station providers, and patients and provide recommendations for strengthening these ties in order to improve care for service members with mild to moderate TBI. Through surveys, site visits, and interviews, we examined the interactions between the NICoE, home station providers responsible for referring patients and implementing NICoE treatment plans, and the service members who receive care.

The aims of the RAND research team's evaluation were to

- evaluate the process for referring service members from the home station to the NICoE
- examine the NICoE assessment and treatment processes, including interactions with the home station during that time
- evaluate the patient's process of transitioning back to the home station and home station providers' implementation of the NICoE recommendations.

Our approach to achieving these aims was to examine the interactions between the NICoE and home stations from three perspectives: (1) providers and staff at the NICoE, (2) home station providers, and (3) service members with mild to moderate TBI and psychological health conditions and their families. The results allowed us to develop a series of recommendations for the NICoE as it seeks to better meet the needs of the population it serves and as it moves forward with its plan to open satellite facilities across the country.

This evaluation focused on the interactions between the NICoE, home station providers, and the service members who receive care. We note that the NICoE is involved in many other activities, such as research and educational activities and the development of satellite clinics, which were outside the scope of this evaluation. Further, we note that this evaluation did not focus on the effectiveness of the NICoE in improving patient outcomes nor on the cost-effectiveness of the NICoE model, both of which are worthy of investigation in the future.

Findings

Home Station Provider Perceptions of the NICoE

Overall, we found that home station providers and patients perceived the NICoE as mitigating some of the barriers service members face in seeking treatment for TBI or psychological health problems, including resource constraints, stigma, and provider turnover at home station facilities. There were differences in how home station providers viewed the role of the NICoE's diagnostic services, however. Providers at smaller, more rural sites viewed the NICoE's clinical role as extremely valuable. Providers from larger facilities were more likely to perceive the NICoE's role as duplicative or equivalent in quality. That said, most providers agreed that more communication and a better understanding of the NICoE's mission and services would help improve coordination among the facilities and providers involved with a patient's care.

Perceptions of the NICoE Referral Process

According to the NICoE, to be eligible for a stay at the NICoE, service members must meet the following criteria:

- Active-duty service member from any service branch (including the National Guard and reservists on orders)
- A mission-related mild or moderate TBI
- A comorbid psychological health condition(s)
- Failure to respond to TBI and mental health care offered at the service member's home station
- The potential and desire to return to duty.

The most common reasons for referring a service member to the NICoE, as reported by home station providers who had made such referrals, were that the patient's TBI or psychological health problems were complex and severe and that the patient's symptoms were not improving with the current treatment. These indicators are consistent with the NICoE's eligibility criteria. However, home station providers also reported referring patients who were undergoing medical evaluations as part of the process for separating from the military and were unlikely to return to full duty. The most commonly endorsed reasons for not referring a patient to the NICoE were that the patient did not have TBI and a co-occurring psychological diagnosis, he or she was responding well to the treatment the clinician was providing, or he or she did not have the capacity to engage safely in an outpatient setting.

While home station providers did not cite lack of access to adequate treatment at the patient's home station as a reason for referral, many former NICoE patients in our survey expressed low levels of satisfaction with the care received at their home station. During site visits, both patients and home station providers noted that patients often faced challenges accessing care, such as long wait times for appointments and staff shortages, and that many patients did not have access to complementary and alternative medicine (CAM) treatment modalities.

In general, the home station providers with whom we spoke during our site visits reported that the referral process was relatively easy, though some providers expressed a desire to have more information from the NICoE about the eligibility criteria and reasons why patients are or are not accepted into the program, to help inform future referrals. Overall, almost all patients who are referred to the NICoE accept the referral.

Perceptions of the NICoE Assessment and Treatment Processes

Our survey and site visit interviews included several questions about provider, patient, and family member satisfaction with the services provided during a patient's stay at the NICoE and the quality of communication between home station providers and NICoE staff. While opinions of the value of a stay at the NICoE, the facility's care model, and its efforts to involve family members in patient care were positive, some providers noted gaps in the NICoE's communication about patient progress to providers and limited knowledge of the services available at home station facilities.

Despite a generally positive impression of NICoE services, home station providers noted a number of concerns. Some providers—particularly those at well-resourced military treatment facilities (MTFs)—did not perceive a significant difference between the types of services offered at the home station and those offered at the NICoE. Other home station providers expressed concern that the NICoE assessment process can appear to question the competency of home station providers by repeating diagnostic assessments that had already been completed. They noted that this practice could contribute to lower levels of patient satisfaction with home station care.

The NICoE places a significant emphasis on education and the opportunity for family members to be informed and involved in a patient's care. Patients and their spouses had generally positive impressions of the NICoE's efforts in this area. We heard some suggestions from patients and their spouses that communication could be improved prior to patients' admission to the NICoE, with more information about what to expect during the stay and a more clearly defined role for family members who accompany patients. Overall, patients and their spouses who participated in our interviews believed that the NICoE's value was in the personal attention provided to patients by a team of providers, the ability to develop integrated and individualized treatment plans that take into account multiple problems, and the flexibility of the treatment options provided.

Experience of Transitioning Back to the Home Station

At the end of a patient's stay at the NICoE, NICoE staff develop an individualized treatment plan with recommendations for follow-up care. The NICoE's diagnostic findings and recommendations are described in a discharge summary intended to direct the treatment the patient will receive when he or she returns to the home station.

During our visit to the NICoE, we learned that the discharge planning process requires collaboration between the interdisciplinary team of NICoE providers and case managers, the home station providers and case manager, and the patient and his or her family. Many home station providers had positive things to say about these opportunities to discuss the NICoE's recommendations and treatment plan.

While some former NICoE patients experienced smooth transitions back to their home stations, others encountered challenges. Several patients recommended better preparation and communication between the two sets of providers and the patient to ensure that the NICoE's recommendations were understood. Home station providers generally agreed that the discharge summary was extremely thorough, though this was not always viewed as a positive. Some home station providers expressed frustration with the length and contents of the summary, and many recommended shortening the summary document and increasing communication between the NICoE and home station providers.

During interviews with NICoE staff and administrators, it appeared that little information is returned to the NICoE about what recommendations are or are not implemented by home station providers. NICoE staff worried about this information void and the possibility that they might be recommending care that the patient would not be able to access, such as CAM therapies that are not readily available in all areas. Indeed, we found that many patients were unable to access CAM treatment at their home stations, and some had difficulty accessing even traditional specialty care.

NICoE patients return home to a variety of treatment facilities. Given the diversity of home stations, it is perhaps not unexpected that satisfaction with home station care also varied. During interviews with former NICoE patients, some noted exceptional care on return to their home stations, and others were dissatisfied with home station services relative to the care they received at the NICoE.

Study Limitations

It is important to consider the limitations of our study when interpreting its conclusions. In particular, there are some limitations to the generalizability of our findings. We did not survey or interview all former NICoE patients and their providers, and, thus, our sample may not be representative of the overall population of former NICoE patients and their providers. The response rates to our survey were only 20–30 percent, though this is in the expected range for web-based surveys. Similarly, we visited a limited number of home stations, and although we sought to maximize variability in experiences with the NICoE with our method of site selection, there may be opinions and experiences not represented in our evaluation. Furthermore, our data collection focused on providers and patients with some familiarity or experience with the NICoE. We cannot speculate on the extent to which our findings about home station TBI care generalize to service members and care providers who lack experience with the NICoE. It is also possible that the overall positive views about the NICoE expressed by former NICoE patients were biased by patients' pretreatment expectations that the NICoE would provide higher quality care than their home station. In particular, these positive expectancies could be due to a perception that more care is better care (Carman et al., 2010). In addition, the study relied on retrospective, self-report methods. Any participant may have recall difficulties, but patients with TBI-related memory impairments may have particular difficulty accurately recalling past experiences. Future evaluations should implement prospective, longitudinal designs to more rigorously assess service members' transitions to and from the NICoE. Still, the surveys and site visits provided rich, detailed information that may contribute to improved care for service members with TBI.

Finally, although the NICoE has become relatively well known among TBI providers and the general public, it had only been operational for four years at the time of this writing and has likely changed a great deal since its inception. It is possible that relationships and communication strategies between the NICoE and home stations have been streamlined and adjusted over time, and our findings do not necessarily account for such adaptations.

Despite these limitations, we believe the integration of multiple data sources, both quantitative and qualitative, provides key insights about communication patterns between NICoE and the home station providers and patient transitions between facilities.

Recommendations

We drew on key findings from the evaluation to develop four categories of recommendations to improve future care for service members with TBI: the NICoE's mission, the process of referring patients to the NICoE, the assessment and treatment services the NICoE provides, and the process by which patients transition back to their home stations.

The NICoE's Mission

Recommendation 1. Clearly define and communicate the clinical, research, and educational roles of the NICoE within the Military Health System (MHS). The NICoE's mission is to play a role in complex TBI treatment, research, and education, but for some NICoE staff and home station providers we spoke with, the role of the NICoE was not yet clear. We identified two specific recommendations in this area.

Recommendation 1a. Review and adapt the NICoE's strategic plan as the NICoE and the MHS evolve. In reviewing and considering revisions of the NICoE's strategic plan, stakeholders should consider the history of the NICoE, the changing context of the MHS, and an articulated vision for the NICoE over the next five or ten years. The strategic plan should also identify measurable goals for the NICoE, with a clear strategy for meeting those goals.

Recommendation 1b. Develop a consistent message about the role of the NICoE and disseminate this message widely. Once the optimal role for the NICoE is determined, the NICoE should clearly, broadly, and routinely disseminate its message about its role, as well as any changes to its policies and how it interacts with service members and home station providers. A strategic plan could be used as a guiding document for developing outreach and messaging materials. Other DoD organizations with similar goals (e.g., DCoE, Defense and Veterans Brain Injury Center [DVBIC]) should work with the NICoE to communicate with stakeholders about the NICoE's role.

Recommendation 2. Foster a collaborative culture between the NICoE and home station providers. Some home station providers felt that their patients returned from the NICoE with a lower opinion of the care they received at their home stations. NICoE and home station providers may have different treatment philosophies and models of care. However, they should work together to develop a clear and collaborative message about the roles of the NICoE and the home station.

Referral of Service Members to the NICoE

Recommendation 3. Inform home station providers about the NICoE's eligibility criteria. We identified three specific recommendations in this area.

Recommendation 3a. List and regularly update eligibility criteria on the NICoE referral form and website. Home station providers expressed confusion about the NICoE's inclusion and exclusion criteria. Eligibility criteria should be clearly stated on the NICoE referral form and on the NICoE website.

Recommendation 3b. Reconsider "potential and desire to return to active duty" as a NICoE eligibility criterion. This criterion appears to be in conflict with other eligibility criteria and does not seem to be consistently implemented, as many NICoE patients reported being in the process of a Medical Evaluation Board review prior to and while at the NICoE. From a force strength perspective, it may be important to restrict access to the NICoE to only those service members who are most likely to return to active duty. If this is the priority, potentially conflicting eligibility criteria may need to be eliminated or revised for clarity.

Recommendation 3c. Adhere to eligibility criteria consistently and clearly communicate to home station providers the rationale for any exceptions or modifications. Eligibility criteria may evolve as the NICoE satellites open and as the needs of service members and the MHS change over time. The NICoE should ensure that its intake and referral processes are as consistent, fair, and transparent as possible. When exceptions or revisions to eligibility criteria must be made, their rationale should be clearly communicated with home station providers.

Recommendation 4. Focus patient recruitment on service members in greatest need. We identified two specific recommendations in this area.

Recommendation 4a. Actively seek referrals for service members at low-resource home stations. Our findings suggest that the patients and providers who perceived the greatest benefit of the NICoE were those located at sites with few resources and who were geographically isolated from major hospitals and treatment centers. Outreach to a wider variety of providers and service members may bring referrals and simultaneously help connect underserved service members with the TBI care they need. In addition to direct patient recruitment, NICoE outreach could include education about the NICoE and its services and consultation with home station providers. If this recommendation is implemented, it will be important to carefully tailor the treatment plan for service members at these sites to ensure the availability of recommended care once they return to their home stations. In addition, unlike patients from high resource stations, these patients may not have completed first-line clinical practice guideline (CPG) recommended treatments for TBI and comorbid mental health conditions (VA/DoD, 2009a; 2009b; 2010). Treatment plans should therefore focus on obtaining evidence-based care for these patients, as opposed to the alternative treatments that are more appropriate for those who have already tried and failed first-line care.

Recommendation 4b. In deciding which patients to accept at the NICoE, consider prioritizing service members who have very complex presentations or who have exhausted all home station treatment options. To conserve resources, the NICoE should consider a more conservative intake process, limiting referrals from high-resource home stations to only the most complex cases and those who have exhausted local treatment options. The NICoE could also offer consultation to home station providers treating patients with complex symptoms in need of certain expertise or a second opinion as a first step before accepting these patients into the NICoE.

NICoE Assessment and Treatment Services
Recommendation 5. Evaluate the effects of NICoE assessment and treatment services on patient outcomes. Future studies using experimental designs or matched comparison groups may help to determine the extent to which NICoE services result in improved patient outcomes compared with treatment as usual.

Recommendation 5a. Conduct a cost analysis of the NICoE. Because the NICoE represents a considerable investment of resources, an analysis should be conducted to determine the costs associated with providing services to service member populations at the NICoE compared with home stations and to identify which services could be provided at home stations for the same or lower cost. We note that any cost analysis should take into account the unique nature of the NICoE as a public-private partnership.

Transitioning from the NICoE Back to the Home Station

Recommendation 6. Increase and formalize communication and coordination between the NICoE and home station providers. We identified two specific recommendations in this area.

Recommendation 6a. Bolster communication and coordination early on in the treatment process (ideally at intake) and sustain this level throughout the patient's stay at the NICoE. Currently, the NICoE communicates with the referring home station provider primarily at intake and discharge and not as much throughout the patient's stay at the NICoE. To improve communication, the NICoE may wish to coordinate the time of these calls with home station providers' schedules to increase the likelihood that the home station provider can attend.

Recommendation 6b. Enhance communication between the NICoE and home station specialty providers. Given that the NICoE is unusual in its integrated interdisciplinary approach to care, we suggest connecting specialists with one another. Improved information sharing may also allow the NICoE to ensure that all treating home station providers—not just the referring provider—are invited to the discharge conference call and directly sent the discharge summary.

Recommendation 7. Streamline discharge summaries and provide recommendations in the context of the treatment already delivered by the home station. We identified two specific recommendations in this area.

Recommendation 7a. List treatment recommendations near the beginning of the report. Several patients and providers noted the NICoE discharge summary is somewhat cumbersome due to its length. They mentioned that the summary would be more helpful if there were a "bottom line up front." For instance, recommendations could be listed on the first page rather than the last page.

Recommendation 7b. Ensure that discharge summaries clearly acknowledge services previously delivered and provide a rationale. Home station providers noted that NICoE treatment recommendations sometimes suggested treatment modes that have already been completed or were ineffective. These providers were uncertain as to whether this was because NICoE providers were unaware of the services previously delivered or because they believed more of that treatment—or a different version of it—would be helpful. In such cases, NICoE providers should explicitly acknowledge previous treatment when they are aware of it and explain the reasoning for suggesting more of the same intervention.

Recommendation 8. Ensure that service members can access recommended care at or near their home station and are aware of its cost. The CAM approaches offered by the NICoE were commonly recommended but often difficult to access at service members' home stations. Before completing the discharge summary, the NICoE should work with the patient and with home station providers to determine (1) whether specific services are available at or near the home station and (2) whether they are covered by the service member's insurance. When a treatment is not covered or easily accessible, the team should prepare a backup plan.

Recommendation 9. Enhance patient tracking and follow-up after discharge. According to participating NICoE staff members, the NICoE aims to follow all of its patients indefinitely after they are discharged to determine whether treatment gains are sustained and whether patients are accessing needed care, as well as to identify gaps in services or barriers to care that must be addressed. To successfully follow the growing number of NICoE patients after discharge and to identify barriers to care and gaps in services, more resources must be invested in this effort, in terms of both manpower and devising a better method for patient follow-up.

Acknowledgments

We gratefully acknowledge the support of our current and previous project monitors at the Defense Centers of Excellence for Psychological Health and Traumatic Brain Injury, Mr. Yoni Tyberg, CAPT John Golden, and Col Christopher Robinson. We also acknowledge the support of individuals at the National Intrepid Center of Excellence, in particular CAPT Sara Kass, Dr. Tom DeGraba, Dr. James Kelly, CDR Wendy Pettit, CAPT Richard Bergthold, and Ms. Kathy Thorp. We appreciate the comments provided by our reviewers, Dr. Kimberly Hepner and Dr. Lisa Brenner. Their constructive critiques were addressed, as part of RAND's rigorous quality assurance process, to improve the quality of this report. We acknowledge the support and assistance of Lisa Miyashiro, Eric Pedersen, Gina Boyd, and Anna Smith in the preparation of this report. We are also grateful to the service members, families, and providers who participated in components of this evaluation for their time, and to our points of contact at each home station for their time and support in facilitating the site visits.

Abbreviations

AHLTA	Armed Forces Health Longitudinal Technology Application
CAM	complementary and alternative medicine
CPAP	continuous positive airway pressure
CPG	clinical practice guideline
DCoE	Defense Centers of Excellence for Psychological Health and Traumatic Brain Injury
DoD	U.S. Department of Defense
DVBIC	Defense and Veterans Brain Injury Center
GED	general educational development
IED	improvised explosive device
IFHF	Intrepid Fallen Heroes Fund
MDD	major depressive disorder
MHS	Military Health System
MTF	military treatment facility
NCO	noncommissioned officer
NICoE	National Intrepid Center of Excellence
NIH	National Institutes of Health
OEF	Operation Enduring Freedom
OIF	Operation Iraqi Freedom
PCM	primary care manager
PCP	primary care provider
PH	psychological health
POC	point of contact

PTSD   posttraumatic stress disorder

SD   standard deviation

SOP   standard operating procedure

TBI   traumatic brain injury

VA   U.S. Department of Veterans Affairs

CHAPTER ONE

Introduction

Between 2001 and 2011, 2.2 million U.S. service members were deployed in support of Operation Enduring Freedom (OEF) and Operation Iraqi Freedom (OIF) (Sayer, 2011). In an era of an all-volunteer force, the pace and demands of these conflicts have resulted in longer and more frequent deployments, and historically high levels of participation by reserve forces (Hosek, Kavanagh, and Miller, 2006; DoD, 2007). Although most service members cope well with deployment-related stresses, the wartime risks of the past decade have resulted in significant rates of physical injuries and psychological health problems among service members (Schell and Marshall, 2008).

Improvised explosive devices (IEDs) have been used extensively against U.S. forces during these conflicts and have been one of the leading causes of death and injury. Those who survive an IED blast often incur a traumatic brain injury (TBI), which has been called the signature injury of the OEF/OIF conflict (Riccitiello, 2010). TBIs can also result from training accidents, motor vehicle accidents, and other traumas, and in fact, non–deployment-related accidents accounted for the bulk of all TBIs in 2013 (DVBIC, 2014).

Neither TBI nor psychological health disorders are necessarily permanent. Many individuals with these conditions experience remission of cognitive and affective symptoms over time and return to baseline functioning (Perkonigg et al., 2005; Schretlen and Shapiro, 2003). Although recovery can occur without formal care, other service members benefit from formal

---

Traumatic Brain Injury (TBI): A traumatically induced structural injury and/or physiological disruption of brain function as a result of an external force that is indicated by new onset or worsening of at least one of the following clinical signs, immediately following the event:

- Any period of loss of or a decreased level of consciousness
- Any loss of memory for events immediately before or after the injury
- Any alteration in mental state at the time of the injury (confusion, disorientation, slowed thinking, etc.)
- Neurological deficits (weakness, loss of balance, change in vision, praxis, paresis/plegia, sensory loss, aphasia, etc.) that may or may not be transient
- Intracranial lesion.

SOURCE: VA/DoD Clinical Practice Guidelines for Management of Concussion/mTBI (2009)

---

diagnostics, assessment, and treatment to help them to regain their original capabilities and return to full duty. For those for whom a full recovery and return to duty is not feasible, these same services can help them to adjust to their new baseline and effectively transition out of the service. While the military health care system has adjusted to meet the unique needs of service members recovering from OEF/OIF physical and mental injuries, not all patients can be optimally served by the standard infrastructure of military treatment facilities. A small proportion of these patients may benefit from specialty services designed to treat TBI and comorbid psychological health conditions.

In response to this need for specialty services, the U.S. Department of Defense (DoD) opened the National Intrepid Center of Excellence (NICoE) in Bethesda, Maryland, in 2010. The NICoE provides interdisciplinary diagnostic evaluations, short-term treatment, and treatment planning for TBI and comorbid psychological health conditions with the goal of supporting service members' ability to continue full service. Service members from across the country travel to the NICoE for a four-week stay, where they receive specialized assessments and individualized treatment plans and then return to their home bases, where local providers coordinate with the NICoE to implement these treatment plans. The NICoE facility accepts five new patients per week, for a total of 20 patients per month. At the time of this evaluation, approximately 400 service members had received services at the NICoE.

Epidemiology of TBI

The annual number of active-duty service members diagnosed with TBI by a medical professional has grown from 12,407 in 2002 to a high of 32,625 in 2011 (DVBIC, 2014). As high as these frequencies may seem, the rate of diagnosed TBIs likely underestimates the true prevalence, as many service members do not seek or receive medical services for their injuries. Population-level surveys of service members provide additional data and estimates of TBI that do not rely on receipt of treatment. In a RAND study of service members previously deployed to OIF/OEF, 19.5 percent reported an injury during their most recent deployment that resulted in an alteration of consciousness—that is, a likely TBI (Schell and Marshall, 2008). Members of the Army or Marine Corps, men, enlisted personnel, and younger service members are more likely to report having experienced a TBI during deployment (Schell and Marshall, 2008) due to the fact that these groups are more likely to have had exposure to combat trauma (Schell and Marshall, 2008).

Severity, Symptoms, and Clinical Course of TBI

The severity of a TBI is graded according to the nature of the trauma and the immediate clinical signs. A mild TBI, also known as a concussion, is diagnosed if alterations in consciousness last no longer than 24 hours; there is either no loss of consciousness or, if present, loss of consciousness lasts no longer than 30 minutes; there is no amnesia or it resolves in less than 24 hours; and motor, verbal, and eye-opening responses remain relatively unimpaired immediately following the trauma (American Congress of Rehabilitation Medicine, 1993; VA, 2010; Teasdale et al., 1979; VA and DoD, 2009). Moderate TBIs are marked by an altered mental state extending to more than 24 hours; a loss of consciousness between 30 minutes and 24 hours; amnesia lasting between one and seven days; and impaired motor, verbal and eye opening responses immediately following the trauma. Severe TBIs are marked by an altered mental state extending to more than 24 hours; a loss of consciousness extending more than 24 hours; amnesia lasting more than seven days; and impaired motor, verbal and eye opening responses immediately following the trauma. Among service members diagnosed with a TBI in 2012, approximately 86 percent were classified as mild (DVBIC, 2012).

TBI symptoms vary significantly depending on the brain regions affected by the trauma. Most patients with TBI will experience some, but rarely all, of the following common symptoms: headache, confusion, agitation, slurred speech, fatigue, sleep disturbances, vestibular disturbances, weakness, sensory problems, memory and concentration difficulties, problems with judgment and executive control, mood changes, irritability, impulsivity, aggression, vomiting/nausea, convulsions, or seizures (VA, 2010; Helmick et al., 2006; McCrea et al., 2009). It is important to note that the severity rating of a TBI is determined by the severity of the immediate response to the trauma, and *not* to the severity of ongoing symptoms (VA, 2010; Helmick et al., 2006; McCrea et al., 2009). Thus, some service members with mild TBIs may experience persistent and debilitating symptoms, while some service members with moderate TBIs may recover quickly and fully. Note as well that the severity diagnosis is not updated over time. A service member with a moderate TBI is not reclassified as a mild TBI as symptoms resolve, but rather retains the original moderate TBI diagnosis (VA, 2010; Helmick et al., 2006; McCrea et al., 2009).

Symptoms associated with mild TBI are typically temporary (Carroll et al., 2004). Eighty-five to 95 percent of civilian patients with a mild TBI can expect a full recovery, very often within one to two weeks of the trauma (Carroll et al., 2004; McCrea et al., 2009; Ruff, 2005). For military service members who screen positive for a mild TBI, 85–90 percent recover within three months (VA, 2010). Without appropriate medical and psychosocial support, the remaining 10–15 percent may experience difficulty with occupational, family, and social reintegration, depression and anxiety, and may isolate themselves from family and friends (VA, 2010). Degree of recovery from moderate and severe TBIs is highly variable and unpredictable. Some patients will experience rapid return to baseline function, while others must learn strategies to adjust to permanent changes in functioning (VA, 2010).

Comorbidity of TBI and Psychiatric Disorders

Compared to service members who have never experienced a TBI, those who have are more likely to develop a psychiatric disorder such as posttraumatic stress disorder (PTSD) or depression. In a survey of previously deployed service members, overall rates of probable PTSD (13.8 percent) and probable depression (13.7 percent) were high, but they were considerably higher among those with a TBI (Schell and Marshall, 2008). Thirty-five percent of service members who had experienced a TBI during their deployment had probable PTSD, and 34 percent had probable depression (Schell and Marshall, 2008). Similarly, in a survey of previously deployed Army soldiers, 44 percent of soldiers who suffered an injury with a loss of consciousness met diagnostic criteria for PTSD, while only 16 percent of soldiers with other types of injuries met diagnostic criteria for PTSD (Hoge et al., 2008). In the same sample, 23 percent of soldiers who lost consciousness following an injury met diagnostic criteria for major depression, while only 7 percent of soldiers with other types of injuries met diagnostic criteria for depression (Hoge et al., 2008).

There are a number of potential explanations for the high rates of comorbidity between TBI and psychiatric conditions, such as PTSD and depression. First, there is significant overlap in the symptom profiles of these conditions. For example, sleep disturbances, fatigue, irritability, alterations in arousal and difficulty concentrating can be associated with all of these conditions, and, as such, having any one disorder may make it easier to meet the diagnostic threshold for others. It is partially for this reason that the diagnostic process for service members with comorbid conditions must be skilled and careful. Second, the precipitating event may lead to both syndromes. That is, an IED blast can both physically injure the brain and also be re-experienced psychologically, resulting in symptoms such as traumatic nightmares or persistent feelings of fear, horror, or anger (among the necessary conditions for PTSD as diagnosed in the Diagnostic and Statistical Manual of Mental Disorders, Fifth Edition [DSM-V]; APA, 2013). Although this may explain some of the overlap between conditions, research by Hoge and colleagues (2008) showed that non-TBI injuries did not predict PTSD to the same degree as TBI, suggesting that the explanation may require more than the simple convergence of injury event and the development of psychological symptoms. Finally, some investigators have suggested that brain areas, such as the orbital prefrontal cortex and related circuitry (e.g., thalamus, basal ganglia), are both particularly vulnerable to the biomechanical forces leading to injury and potentially critical to neurobehavioral regulation leading to risk for PTSD and depression (Stein and McAllister, 2009). This hypothesis requires additional research, however.

The NICoE Program

To address the complex needs of service members with mild to moderate TBI and comorbid psychological health conditions, the NICoE is designed around an interdisciplinary approach to assessment and treatment (NICoE, 2014a). Providers from different disciplines are housed under one roof and meet to share information regularly. Patients at the NICoE stay for four weeks, receiving intensive diagnostic and assessment services (NICoE, 2014c). During this time, the service member should receive a tailored approach to diagnostic evaluation and other assessments in a patient-centered environment (NICoE, 2014c). The diagnostic equipment at the NICoE includes advanced neuroimaging tools such as magnetic resonance imaging (MRI) and magnetoencephalography (MEG) that are often difficult to access in usual care settings but have the potential to assist in the diagnosis of complex cases (NICoE, 2014a). Other resources include the Computer Assisted Rehabilitation Environment (CAREN), a technical system that can test service members' agility and motor skills in a virtual environment (e.g., a virtual combat zone, or the driver's seat of a car) (De Groot et al., 2003).

Over the course of four weeks, each patient meets with a variety of care providers as needed, representing as many as 16 different disciplines, which can include an art therapist, audiologist, chaplain, licensed clinical social worker, neurologist, neuropsychologist, nutrition specialist, occupational therapist, optometrist, physical therapist, psychiatrist, recreational therapist, sleep medicine physician, speech and language pathologist, and others (NICoE, 2014b). Other services include rehabilitation through the use of a motion simulator, driving simulator, or firearms simulator, and Complementary and Alternative Medicine (CAM) approaches such as yoga and acupuncture (NICoE, 2014a; NICoE, 2014b). Service members can also participate in the NICoE's canine program, where patients are encouraged to interact with and train a service animal (NICoE, 2014a). Patient and family education curricula focused on empowerment and self-advocacy are also available (NICoE, 2014b).

The NICoE provides short-term treatment for TBI and comorbid psychological health conditions and considers these treatments an extension of its assessment mission. That is, the four-week stay provides an opportunity for the patient to "try out" new treatment approaches, but the stay is not sufficiently long to provide a full course of treatment. Those treatments that the patient and provider perceive to be beneficial during this assessment period are added to the patient's long-term treatment plan. Most of the evaluated treatments (e.g., acupuncture, art therapy) are not included as recommended treatments in the Department of Veterans Affairs (VA) and DoD's joint clinical practice guidelines (CPGs) for TBI, PTSD, or major depressive disorder (MDD; VA/DoD 2009a; 2009b; 2010), and NICoE providers did not indicate that their treatment approaches are guided by CPGs during our site visit. We see three potential explanations for the lack of reliance on CPGs to guide evidence-based care. First, NICoE administrators and providers may devalue standardized approaches to care for patients with complex medical and psychological needs. Alternatively, providers may know or believe that evidence-based treatments have already been tried by home station providers and failed, and thus appropriately prioritize secondary approaches. Finally, NICoE administrators and providers may value the evaluation of untested strategies as part of the center's research agenda. An assessment of the NICoE's philosophy with respect to CPGs to determine the most likely reason(s) for limited attention to CPG recommendations was outside the scope of this evaluation.

Each patient's experience at the NICoE begins with an intake appointment where all providers gather to hear the patient's story, helping to ensure that patients are not required to convey the same information to many different providers. After a service member has received a full evaluation by the interdisciplinary NICoE care team over the four-week stay, a discharge report is compiled with diagnostic findings and an individualized treatment plan (NICoE, 2014a). The treatment plan is designed for the providers at the service member's home station to implement. These processes are described in more detail in Chapters Four through Six.

Overview of the NICoE Evaluation

The evolution of the NICoE is atypical within the Military Health System (MHS). Rather than growing from an existing TBI or mental health clinic to become a Center of Excellence, the NICoE was developed from the ground up. Although it necessarily commenced care with no history in the MHS, it was expected to integrate quickly into a large and complex system of care. Moreover, its charter was to take an immediate leadership role in facilitating the implementation of effective treatment for service members when they returned to their home stations. Such transitions between providers have been shown to increase risk for treatment delays and medical errors, and improving care transitions reduces health care costs (Eslami and Tran, 2014; Gardner et al., 2014; Tomaszewski et al., 2014). Illustrating the significance of transitions to care, the Affordable Care Act funded the Community-based Care Transitions Program to mitigate such risks by implementing evidence-based care transition interventions at hospital discharge (Daughtridge, Archibald, and Conway, 2014). Given the complexity of the institutional relationships as patients transition to and from the NICoE, the Center's ability to effectively and efficiently address the needs of service members and their families requires special attention to transition processes. This report evaluates the complex communication and relationships between the NICoE, home station providers, and patients and provides recommendations for strengthening these ties in order to improve care for service members with mild to moderate TBI. An evaluation testing the effectiveness or quality of the NICoE's services was considered but ultimately determined to be unfeasible for two reasons: (1) the study time frame and budget would not accommodate a rigorous evaluation (e.g., a longitudinal study), and (2) NICoE leadership felt that their internal research and evaluation activities already address these areas and thus were not willing to participate in a RAND evaluation that they viewed as redundant.

To evaluate relationships between the NICoE and home station providers, our aims focused on patient transition points and NICoE communication with home station providers. They included (1) evaluation of the process for referring service members from the home station to the NICoE; (2) examination of the NICoE assessment and treatment processes, including interactions with the home station during that time; and (3) evaluation of the patient's process of transitioning back to the home station and home station providers' implementation of the NICoE's recommendations. Our approach to achieving these aims was to examine the interactions between the NICoE and home stations from three perspectives: (1) providers and staff at the NICoE, (2) home station providers, and (3) service members with mild to moderate TBI and psychological health conditions and their families. We drew on these three perspectives in order to identify the full range of factors and circumstances that influence referral to the NICoE and implementation of NICoE recommendations, ultimately providing recommendations to improve the impact of the NICoE within the MHS. These perspectives were obtained through surveys, site visits to the NICoE and other military installations, and interviews with providers, service members and family members. Web-based surveys were conducted with providers and service members who have received services at the NICoE.

Limits of This Evaluation

This evaluation focused on transitions to and from the NICoE. However, the NICoE is involved in many other activities that were outside the scope of the current evaluation. Although the following areas and issues may be referenced within this report, it is important to note that the evaluation does not address them specifically.

1. *Satellite Clinics.* As this evaluation was under way, the NICoE was developing satellite clinics at a number of installations. Since the satellite clinics were not in operation at the time of our evaluation, we do not address the functions of these clinics nor how the role of the "parent" NICoE facility may be changed or influenced as a result of the satellites. In future studies of the NICoE, it will be important to assess the role of satellite clinics with respect to the parent facility, the population of service members they care for, and the utility and effectiveness of the services they provide.
2. *The NICoE's Research Activities.* The NICoE is engaged in research on TBI, but an examination of the Center's research activities and their impact was not possible for this evaluation.

3. *Quality of Care.* The focus of this report was on the quality of communication and patient transitions between the NICoE and home station providers. Although NICoE services are described to provide context, the quality of that care—as defined as consistency with research evidence and clinical practice guidelines—was not systematically assessed.

4. *Patient Outcomes.* An evaluation of the effect of receiving care at the NICoE on patient outcomes (e.g., symptom improvement) would have required time and resources that were not available for this study. The NICoE routinely collects patient outcome data, however, which could be used by the NICoE or outside organizations to determine whether treatment at the NICoE leads to improvement in TBI and other symptoms.

5. *Cost-Effectiveness.* Given the comprehensiveness of the NICoE's program, an evaluation of its cost-effectiveness is worthy of investigation. Unfortunately, however, we were unable to examine cost within the study's time frame and budget.

Organization of This Report

The report is organized into seven chapters. Chapter Two describes the methods and samples used for the evaluation. Chapter Three outlines the history and mission of the NICoE, and subsequent chapters present the study results with regard to the NICoE's referral processes (Chapter Four), the NICoE's diagnostic and treatment processes (Chapter Five), and the processes by which patients are discharged from the NICoE and transition back to their home stations (Chapter Six). Chapter Seven summarizes the study's conclusions and recommendations. The discussion guides for our site visits with NICoE staff, patients, spouses/caregivers, and home station providers can be found in Appendixes A–D, respectively. The provider and patient survey forms can be found in Appendix E.

CHAPTER TWO

Evaluation Methods

The aims of the RAND research team's evaluation of the NICoE were to (1) describe the NICoE's assessment and treatment services; (2) evaluate the process of referral of service members from the home station to the NICoE; (3) examine the NICoE assessment and treatment processes, including interactions with the home station during that time; and (4) evaluate the patient's process of transitioning back to the home station and home station providers' implementation of the NICoE's recommendations.

We examined these systems and processes from three perspectives:

- NICoE staff, including providers
- Home station providers
- Former NICoE patients and their families.

In this chapter, we describe the methods we used to collect data from each perspective. We begin by discussing the procedures, followed by the measures and data analyses. All methods were reviewed and approved by RAND's Human Subjects Protection Committee, as well as the U.S. Army Medical Research and Materiel Command's Office of Research Protections.

Procedures

NICoE Site Visit
We conducted a site visit to the NICoE facility in Bethesda, Maryland, to solicit the perspectives of NICoE staff and administrators. The visit took place over two days in the spring of 2013. Four RAND research staff (two Ph.D. level, two M.A. level) conducted the site visit, which included a review of the NICoE's mission and its clinical, research, and education activities; a tour of the NICoE facility; and group and individual discussions with administrators and providers. No identifying information was collected, and all participating staff provided verbal informed consent.

Home Station Site Visits
To obtain the perspectives of those who provide care to service members with mild to moderate TBI and service members who have been to the NICoE and their spouses,[1] we selected eight military installations for home station site visits based on the following criteria:

---

[1] Although family members other than the patients' spouse (e.g., a parent) are permitted to accompany the patient to the NICoE, nearly all accompanying family members are spouses. For simplicity, for the remainder of the report, we refer to

- Number of referrals to the NICoE
- Branch of service
- Types of units
- Geography and demographics.

To maximize variability, we worked with the NICoE to select some sites that had referred the largest number of service members (high referrers) and others that had referred few service members, despite housing highly combat-exposed units (low referrers). Referral patterns were based on routinely collected referral source data from the NICoE. We opted to select home stations from the Army and Marine Corps, as soldiers and marines have the highest rates of TBI in the U.S. military (Armed Forces Health Surveillance Center, 2012). Similarly, we included sites serving special forces/special operations units, as well as a Warrior Transition Unit serving reserve component combat-exposed service members living in rural locations far from major military installations. For budgetary reasons, we selected only sites within the continental United States.

During the site visits, we conducted individual interviews and focus groups with directors of TBI clinics, TBI providers (e.g., neurologists, psychologists, psychiatrists, occupational therapists, speech therapists, physical therapists, case managers), and service members who had been patients at the NICoE and their spouses. To accommodate former NICoE patients who were unable to meet with us during the scheduled site visit, we offered the option of conducting the interview via telephone. No identifiable or protected health information was collected, and all participants provided verbal informed consent.

Surveys

Since the visited home stations were selected based on criteria that may limit the generalizability of findings, we also conducted two web surveys to obtain a wider variety of perspectives from (1) providers who had referred patients to the NICoE and (2) service members who had received services from the NICoE. Both surveys were launched in September 2013 and were open for approximately two months. Surveys of patient experiences and their satisfaction with care are recommended data sources in process evaluations designed to assess how care is implemented (Hulscher, Laurant, and Grol, 2003). Prior to completing the surveys, all respondents completed informed consent procedures. No identifying information was collected as part of the survey.

Survey of Referring Providers

The NICoE provided the RAND research team with a list of the names and email addresses of providers who had referred one or more patients to the NICoE (N=201). Providers included a mix of civilian and uniformed providers. A RAND researcher sent an invitation email containing a link to the confidential survey to all providers. For email invitations that were returned undelivered, we searched the DoD global address list to find alternate email addresses. Ultimately, the invitation was sent successfully to a total of 184 referring providers (92 percent of the original list supplied by the NICoE). Of the remaining providers, two (1 percent) had retired (as indicated by automated email reply), and we were unable to find valid email addresses for 15

---

patients' spouses.

(7 percent). Three reminder emails to encourage participation were sent at two-week intervals following the initial invitation.

Survey of Former NICoE Patients

To maintain the confidentiality of NICoE patients, we did not obtain patient contact information. Instead, NICoE staff forwarded an email invitation from RAND to all former NICoE patients (N=369) for the NICoE patient survey. Emails to 16 percent (n=58) of the former NICoE patients were returned undeliverable, resulting in 311 successfully delivered emails. The invitation contained a link to the anonymous survey. The NICoE forwarded email reminders to patients two and four weeks after the initial email invitation.

Measures

NICoE Site Visit

Confidential interviews with NICoE staff covered referral and intake processes; assessment, treatment, and monitoring of the patient at the NICoE; and discharge, treatment planning, and patient follow-up. We also asked administrators about the overall mission of the NICoE. The RAND research team generated semi-structured interview guides to help guide the discussion within these areas (Appendix A).

Home Station Site Visits

We designed separate semi-structured interview guides for site directors, providers, service members, and service members' spouses to be used at the home station site visits (Appendixes B–D). These interviews were also confidential.

Site directors (e.g., director of the TBI clinic) were asked about the services their site offers to TBI patients, their perception of the NICoE, and experiences referring to the NICoE and receiving patients back from the NICoE. At home stations with a planned NICoE satellite, we also asked about how referral processes and post-NICoE care are expected to change once the satellite clinic is in operation.

We asked providers about their professional background, knowledge about the NICoE, their experiences referring patients to the NICoE, and their experiences working with the NICoE and the patient through treatment planning, discharge, and upon the patient's return to the home station. For providers who had not interacted with patients who went to the NICoE, we asked about their understanding of the NICoE, as well as the influences on their decision (not) to refer a patient to the NICoE.

Service members who had been patients at the NICoE and their spouses were asked questions about the TBI assessment and treatment they received before, during, and after the NICoE. To enable us to determine how the former NICoE patients we spoke with might be similar to or different from other NICoE patients, we asked them to complete a short questionnaire assessing age, gender, race and ethnicity, marital status, military status, year they joined the service, service branch, and pay grade. Family members were also asked to categorize their relationship to the NICoE patient (husband/wife, parent, grandparent, brother/sister, adult child, other). Because nearly all family members were the spouses of NICoE patients, for the remainder of the report we refer to this group as *spouses*. Few spouses participated (N=4).

Surveys

The referring provider and NICoE patient surveys were developed using existing measures showing acceptable levels of reliability and validity in previously published studies whenever possible. However, to reduce survey length, some scales were abbreviated. Where necessary, items were adapted for the military context. In domains where no existing measures were available (e.g., reasons a provider would or would not refer a patient to the NICoE) RAND researchers generated items. Wherever possible, RAND-generated items use response options similar or identical to those used in previously published scales. Appendix E includes a description of the measures that were used in each survey.

The *referring provider survey* contained two screening questions verifying that the provider had heard of the NICoE and that the provider sees patients with TBI or psychological health conditions and 58 additional survey items. Eligible providers completed items assessing demographics (e.g., education, military status) and practice characteristics (experience treating patients with TBI and co-occurring psychological health disorders). Other survey domains included providers' familiarity with the NICoE (e.g., number of patients referred to the NICoE), referral decisions (e.g., "I would refer a patient to the NICoE if…" [check all that apply among seven response options]), and experience treating patients who had been discharged from the NICoE (e.g., satisfaction with and usefulness of the NICoE's treatment recommendations).

The *patient survey* began with a screening question to verify the respondent had been to the NICoE, followed by 72 additional survey items. The survey included demographic questions (e.g., gender, age) and items about the care received before, during, and after the NICoE (e.g., satisfaction, treatment barriers, and facilitators).

Data Analyses

Installation and NICoE Site Visits

Installation and NICoE site visit data were pile sorted and coded according to Ryan et al.'s (2009) method of qualitative data analysis. Specifically, site visit notes were divided into segments reflecting a single idea. Note segments were then categorized by source (provider/patient/spouse and site) and the section of the interview in which it appeared (e.g., referral process). These source and section categories were used to provide context to the note segment during the coding process.

One researcher then coded the segments into categories of similar content or "themes," and a second researcher reviewed the coding. In cases in which there was disagreement about a segment code, the researchers met to discuss it and reach consensus. Note segments that fit more than one theme were coded into multiple categories as needed.

Surveys

Provider Survey

We used descriptive statistics (frequencies, means, standard deviations) to summarize the characteristics of providers who refer patients to the NICoE, their familiarity with the NICoE, and their experiences referring to the NICoE as well as seeing patients after discharge.

Patient Survey

We also used descriptive statistics (frequencies, means, standard deviations) to summarize former NICoE patients' demographics; pre-NICoE functioning and TBI care; satisfaction and experience at the NICoE including NICoE treatment recommendations, functioning, and care; and facilitators and barriers to receiving NICoE-recommended care after returning to the home station.

Sample Characteristics

In this section, we briefly describe the site visit and survey participants. First, we describe the individuals who participated in the site visit interviews, where we limit the amount of information provided about participants at each site in order to preserve confidentiality. Then, we discuss the characteristics of the providers and former NICoE patients who participated in the web surveys. Table 2.1 shows the total number of individuals in each group who participated in site visits and the surveys.

NICoE Site Visit

Over the course of two days at the NICoE, we met with approximately 25 NICoE staff through 15 separate individual or group discussions. These included clinical, administrative, and research staff, as well as military and civilian personnel.

Home Station Site Visits

We conducted site visits at eight home stations: Three sites were large active-duty Army installations, one site primarily served U.S. Army Reserve/Army National Guard personnel, two sites were large active-duty Marine Corps installations, and two sites were primarily active-duty Navy installations. Six of the eight sites had a large military medical center with a TBI specialty clinic. One of the sites without a large military medical center had access to a nearby large treatment facility. One site was geographically distant from any large military treatment facility or specialty TBI clinic. (See Table 2.2.) The majority of the sites served a large number of operational units and thus a potentially high number of combat-exposed service members. The total full-time military population of the active-duty home stations visited ranged from approximately 7,000 to more than 50,000.[2]

Table 2.1
Number of Participants, by Data Collection Strategy

Data Collection Strategy	Participants		
	Providers	Former NICoE Patients	Spouses of Former NICoE Patients
NICoE site visit	25	0	0
Home station site visits	71	25	4
Web surveys	56	65	N/A

---

2   Army Stationing and Installation Plan data, 2014; information from installations' public websites, 2014.

Table 2.2
Home Station Installation Site Descriptions

Site Identifier	High or Low Referrer to NICoE	Type of Home Station
Site A	High	No TBI treatment facility; remote home station
Site B	Low	Large treatment facility; low number of operational units and lower potential for combat exposure
Site C	Low	Large treatment facility; high number of operational units and potential for high levels of combat exposure
Site D	Low	Large treatment facility; high number of operational units and potential for high levels of combat exposure
Site E	High	Large treatment facility; high number of operational units and potential for high levels of combat exposure
Site F	Low	Large treatment facility; high number of operational units and potential for high levels of combat exposure
Site G	Low	Large treatment facility; high number of operational units and potential for high levels of combat exposure
Site H	High	Near to large treatment facility; high number of operational units and potential for high levels of combat exposure

NOTES: Installations were categorized as "high" or "low" referrers based on NICoE-provided data and home station reports of usage. "Type of home station" is based on a qualitative description of the TBI and psychological health services on the home station and the patient population served (e.g., large treatment facility, small treatment facility, number of combat-exposed personnel).

Across the seven home station site visits, we spoke with 71 different providers and clinic administrators, 25 former NICoE patients, and four spouses. Demographic information about providers was not collected. Participating former NICoE patients were mostly male (96 percent), white (88 percent), and active duty (88 percent). Sixty percent of the former NICoE patients were married or living with a partner. Most (60 percent) of the former NICoE patients we spoke with were in the Army, 24 percent were in the Marine Corps, and the remainder (16 percent) were in the Navy or Air Force. Sixteen percent held a rank of E1 to E4; 60 percent were E5 to E9; and 20 percent were officers (O1 to O6). Four percent of participants did not answer the rank/pay grade question. The mean age of former NICoE patients was 37 years (standard deviation [SD]=6.7). All participating spouses were female, white, and married to the former NICoE patient. Their mean age was also 37 years (SD=6.6).

NICoE Referring Provider Survey Respondents

Fifty-six of the 184 providers who were invited to participate in the web survey consented to participate (30.4-percent response rate), and two actively refused. One of the 56 consenting providers had never heard of the NICoE, and one did not respond to our screening question about whether the provider sees patients with TBI; these individuals were screened out. Our final sample of provider survey participants included 54 providers who had heard of the NICoE and reported seeing patients with TBI. The demographics and professional background of the provider survey respondents are shown in Table 2.3. The majority (63 percent) of providers had a doctoral-level education. A variety of disciplines were represented in the sample, with primary care being the most frequently occurring specialty (47.2 percent). Nearly half (46.3

Table 2.3
Demographic and Professional Characteristics of Provider Survey Respondents

Characteristic	N (Total=54)	Percentage of Sample
Education level		
Associate's degree or below	0	0.0
Bachelor's	1	1.9
Master's	19	35.2
Doctoral	34	63.0
Primary discipline		
Clinical psychology	9	17.0
Neurology	6	11.3
Neuropsychology	0	0.0
Occupational therapy	0	0.0
Physical therapy	0	0.0
Primary care	25	47.2
Psychiatry	5	9.4
Social work	4	7.5
Speech therapy	1	1.9
Other	3	5.7
Military status		
Active-duty military	25	46.3
Reserve or National Guard	0	0.0
Non-DoD civilian practitioner/ contractor	9	16.7
DoD employee	17	31.5
Retired military	0	0.0
Other	3	5.6
Branch of service		
Air Force	3	5.6
Army	9	16.7
Coast Guard	0	0.0
Marine Corps	0	0.0
Navy	16	29.6
Not applicable	26	48.1

Table 2.3—Continued

Characteristic	N (Total=54)	Percentage of Sample
Rank		
O3	5	17.9
O4	11	39.3
O5	5	17.9
O6	7	25.0
	Mean (SD)	**Min–Max**
Years of experience with TBI patients	8.5 (8.3)	1–46
Percentage of caseload=TBI patients	67.9 (37.2)	1–100

NOTE: SD = Standard deviation; Min = Minimum; Max = Maximum.

percent) of providers were active-duty military personnel, with approximately a third (29.6 percent) from the Navy. Not surprisingly, providers who were also military personnel were officers, and over a third of this group held the rank of O4 (39.3 percent). Providers reported an average of 8.5 (*SD*=8.3) years of experience with TBI patients and estimated that a mean of 68 percent (*SD*=37.2) of their caseload consisted of TBI patients.

The ways in which providers learned about the NICoE are shown in Table 2.4. Providers most commonly reported that they had heard about the NICoE from a colleague (46.3 percent).

The proportions of providers who had referred patients to the NICoE and worked with patients returning from the NICoE are shown in Table 2.5.

NICoE Patient Survey Respondents

Sixty-five of the 311 former NICoE patients who were invited to participate in the web survey consented to participate (21 percent response rate). Three of the 65 consenting individuals denied ever being a patient at the NICoE, so those individuals were screened out. Our final

Table 2.4
How Providers Learned About the NICoE (N=54)

Method	N (percent)
A colleague	25 (46.3)
A patient	2 (3.7)
A research article, publication, or conference presentation	3 (5.6)
A training/workshop	4 (7.4)
My supervisor	9 (16.7)
National or local media	2 (3.7)
Other	8 (14.8)
Missing	1 (1.9)

Table 2.5
Number and Percentage of Providers Who Referred Patients to the NICoE and/or Saw Them After Their Return from the NICoE (N=53)

		Saw Patients After the NICoE	
		Yes	No
Referred Patients to the NICoE	Yes	37 (68.5%)	13 (24.1%)
	No	1 (1.9%)	2 (3.7%)

NOTE: One provider did not respond to these questions, resulting in the N of 53.

sample for the patient survey included 62 respondents who reported having been a patient at the NICoE. The demographic and military background characteristics of the patient survey respondents are shown below in Table 2.6. This table also juxtaposes the characteristics of soldiers who were hospitalized with a TBI-related diagnosis while on deployment to Iraq (N=2,241) or Afghanistan (N=207) between 2001 and 2007 (Wojcik et al., 2010). While our methods are different from this study and include service members from all branches of service, this comparison may provide some information about how generalizable our sample is relative to the larger population of service members with TBI. The majority of respondents to our patient survey were male (95.2 percent), white (82.3 percent), and not Hispanic or Latino (88.7 percent). Survey respondents reported a range of educational levels, though most had completed at least some college coursework. The average age of respondents was 39.6 (SD=9.2). In terms of military background, the majority of former NICoE patients were on active duty (83.9 percent) at the time of the survey. Approximately 45 percent of patient survey respondents said they were neither separated nor in the process of separating from the military for medical reasons. However, 38.7 percent were in the process of separating for medical reasons, and 16.1 percent had already separated for medical reasons. Approximately 45 percent of respondents were in the Army, 25.8 percent in the Navy, 19.4 percent in the Air Force, and 9.7 percent in the Marine Corps. A substantial proportion of the Navy respondents may have been Navy Seals; according to our qualitative findings, the NICoE sees a disproportionately large number of Seals. The majority of respondents were either mid-level or senior noncommissioned officers (NCOs). Respondents estimated they had deployed an average of 4.3 times (SD=3.2) for OIF, OEF, OND, or another contingency.

As seen in Table 2.6, the former NICoE patients we surveyed were similar to the larger comparison population of soldiers with TBI in proportion of males, Hispanics/Latinos, and reservists. Our sample of former NICoE patients, however, has slightly smaller proportions of African American, National Guard, and enlisted service members and appears to be older. Interpretation of any apparent differences is not advised, however. Due to important qualitative differences in these samples (e.g., NICoE intentionally selects patients with more complex presentations; we surveyed across multiple services and not just one), we did not run tests for statistical significance. Unfortunately, we were unable to find published data to help determine the generalizability of our sample of spouses.

Table 2.6
Demographic and Military Characteristics of Patient Survey Respondents and Soldiers Admitted for TBI Diagnosis During Deployment

Characteristic	N (Total=62)	Percentage of total sample	Soldiers admitted for TBI diagnosis during deployment, 2001–2007 (Afghanistan N=207; Iraq N=2,241)
Gender			
Male	59	95.2	97.1–97.5%
Female	3	4.8	2.5–2.9%
Hispanic/Latino			
Yes	7	11.3	10.0–11.1%
No	55	88.7	NR
Race			
White	51	82.3	71.0–72.5%
Black or African American	2	3.2	7.7–12.2%
Asian	1	1.6	NR
Native Hawaiian/Pacific Islander	0	0.0	NR
American Indian/Alaskan Native	0	0.0	NR
Other	1	1.6	0.0–1.3%
More than one race	4	6.5	NR
Missing/unknown	3	4.8	5.4–8.7%
Education			
High school diploma/GED	8	12.9	NR
Some college	16	25.8	NR
Associate's degree	13	21.0	NR
Bachelor's degree	13	21.0	NR
Graduate degree	12	19.4	NR
Status			
Active Duty	52	83.9	75.6–78.7%
Reserve	4	6.5	5.5–6.8%
National Guard	6	9.7	14.5–18.9%
Medically separated			
Not separated or not in process	28	45.2	NR
In process of separating	24	38.7	NR
Already separated	10	16.1	NR

Table 2.6—Continued

Characteristic	N (Total=62)	Percentage of total sample	Soldiers admitted for TBI diagnosis during deployment, 2001–2007 (Afghanistan N=207; Iraq N=2,241)
Service			
Air Force	12	19.4	N/A
Army	28	45.2	100%
Coast Guard	0	0.0	N/A
Marine Corps	6	9.7	N/A
Navy	16	25.8	N/A
Rank			
Junior NCO	3	4.8	Enlisted=89.4–93.6% Officers=6.3–10.1%
Mid-level NCO	25	40.3	
Senior NCO	18	29.0	
Warrant company-grade officer	4	6.5	
Field-grade officer	12	19.4	
	Mean (SD)	**Min–Max**	
Number of deployments	4.3 (3.2)	1–14	NR
Age	39.6 (9.2)	23–63	66.2–69.1%, ages 20–29

SOURCE: Percentage of soldiers admitted for TBI diagnosis during deployment from Wojcik et al., 2010.

NOTE: GED = General Educational Development test; NCO = noncommissioned officer; SD = standard deviation; NR = not reported; N/A = not applicable.

CHAPTER THREE

History and Mission of the NICoE

The first aim of this evaluation was to provide a comprehensive description of the NICoE, including its history, mission, and assessment services. In this chapter, we address this aim by describing the history of the NICoE and, drawing on information obtained during the site visits, we describe the mission and goals of the NICoE, as well as its role within the Military Health System, both from the perspective of NICoE staff and from that of home station providers.

History and Motivation

In 2007, Congress passed the annual National Defense Authorization Act, which required DoD to create centers of excellence to better understand and care for service members with a TBI and a co-occurring psychological health condition as a result of the recent conflicts (Public Law 110-181, 2008). In response to this charge, DoD created the Defense Center of Excellence for Psychological Health and Traumatic Brain Injury (DCoE) in November 2007 (U.S. Government Accountability Office, 2011). DCoE comprised six component centers responsible for training, developing telehealth and technology services, treatment, and research (U.S. Government Accountability Office, 2011). One of these centers was the NICoE.

The NICoE was established as a public-private partnership with contributions through the Intrepid Fallen Heroes Fund (IFHF).[1] The IFHF is an independent, nonprofit organization established to provide support for wounded military personnel and their families. By 2010, IFHF had funded and completed construction of the 72,000-square-foot NICoE facility at Walter Reed National Military Medical Center through private donations totaling approximately $65 million. The building was designed with the symptoms of the patient population in mind, including considerations for some patients' sensitivity to light. The travel and per diem of the service members assigned to the NICoE on temporary duty orders are funded by the service member's home station unit. Service members, and their families if they elect to attend, are lodged in the Fisher House[2] during their temporary duty at the NICoE; this stay is provided at no cost to the service member.

IFHF also has efforts under way to design and build satellite NICoE clinics at nine other military installations across the country: Ft. Belvoir, Virginia; Camp Lejeune, North Carolina;

---

[1] More information about the Intrepid Fallen Heroes Fund can be found on its website, FallenHeroesFund.org.

[2] The Fisher House is funded through the Fisher House Foundation. Additional information can be found on its website, FisherHouse.org.

Camp Pendleton, California; Fort Bragg, North Carolina; Fort Campbell, Kentucky; Fort Hood, Texas; Joint Base Lewis McChord, Washington; Fort Carson, Colorado; and Fort Bliss, Texas. By summer 2013, construction had begun on satellite centers at Ft. Belvoir, Virginia; Camp Lejeune, North Carolina; and Fort Campbell, Kentucky. As noted in Chapter One, at the time of the RAND evaluation, the NICoE satellite clinics were under construction, had not yet opened, and were therefore not included in the evaluation.

The NICoE is physically located on the campus of the Naval Support Activity Bethesda, home of Walter Reed National Military Medical Center in Bethesda, Maryland. The NICoE began seeing patients in October 2010 and, as of January 2013, had served approximately 400 service members representing all branches of service.

The Mission and Goals of the NICoE Program

The stated vision of the NICoE is "to be the nation's institute for traumatic brain injury and psychological health dedicated to advancing science, enhancing understanding, maximizing health, and relieving suffering" (NICoE, 2014d). Its stated mission is to "deliver comprehensive and holistic care, conduct focused research, and export knowledge to benefit service members, their families, and society" (NICoE, 2014d). Thus, in addition to direct patient care, the NICoE's broader mission includes training, educational, and research activities, although an evaluation of those components of its mission was outside of the scope of this study.

The NICoE has described its clinical model as "a model of holistic, interdisciplinary evaluation and treatment in a family focused, collaborative environment that promotes physical, psychological, and spiritual healing of service members with the complex interaction of TBI and PH [psychological health] who are not responding to conventional therapy elsewhere in the Military Health System (MHS)." Although treatment is included in NICoE services, comprehensive assessment is the primary aim. When treatment services are offered, they are conceptualized as a form of assessment. That is, by offering brief introductions to therapies such as art therapy, yoga, and group therapy, the NICoE seeks to determine—in collaboration with the patient—whether these services are acceptable and potentially useful to the patient. Those that are will be included in treatment recommendations for the patient to pursue on return to his or her home station.

Perceptions of the NICoE's Role Within the MHS

As the NICoE is a unique entity within the MHS, understanding its role in relation to existing military treatment facilities (MTFs) is important. During our site visits, both NICoE staff and home station providers expressed a wide range of views about what they thought the NICoE's role was, suggesting that there is a lack of consensus or understanding about the role that the NICoE plays within the MHS.

Most NICoE staff felt that the NICoE's clinical mission and priorities had evolved over the years. There was some disagreement among NICoE staff about whether the center's mission and priorities were clearly defined. In a discussion about the forthcoming NICoE satellite clinics, one staff member remarked that "what NICoE is isn't clearly defined. How can you replicate something that isn't clearly defined?" Similarly, another noted, "There's a lack of education about what our mission and our vision is." There also appeared to be some disagreement about the target patient population, and some staff members commented that the nature of the patient population had changed over time. For example, one respondent felt that the NICoE's mission was to address only the most medically challenging patients:

> We do not have the same patient population as when we opened in 2010. They are much more complicated now. That's what I think our mission is: We get the hardest of the hard.

Some home station providers had no knowledge of the NICoE's role or the clinical services it provided, while others had extensive experience interacting with the NICoE. Among those who were familiar with the NICoE, some thought diagnostic services were the focus, others thought treatment was the focus, and others were uncertain: "We're still trying to figure out 'What purpose does NICoE serve?'" For those who were unsure about the NICoE's role, most agreed that they wanted to learn more about the NICoE and have a collaborative, two-way relationship. "I would like [the NICoE] to reach out to us," said one provider. Many participants expressed interest in learning more about the NICoE's mission and welcomed a briefing from the NICoE or other face-to-face interaction. Some providers expressed an interest in having more regular dialogue with their NICoE counterparts in a certain discipline and suggested that it would be helpful to have providers visit the NICoE and meet with their discipline's team.

However, not all interviewees expressed uncertainty about the NICoE's role within the MHS. Among those who were familiar with the NICoE, there seemed to be consensus that the NICoE's main role was to serve as an assessment and treatment provider for patients whose symptoms are not improving and who need a "fresh start" to treatment.

The NICoE as a Fresh Start for Treatment

NICoE staff members noted that one of the center's assets is that it is a neutral and private location away from the challenges of a service member's daily work responsibilities and personal life. NICoE staff suggested that this "fresh start" away from daily duties increases service members' willingness to actively engage with treatment: "It starts with getting away. It gives us that momentum and that willingness. They're prepped to do the necessary work when they get here."

Some home station providers agreed that the temporary duty time at a new location was a valuable contribution and worth the referral. They mentioned the "spa effect" of the NICoE, which gives patients an opportunity to get away from their daily responsibilities and focus exclusively on their health care. This was one benefit that could not be replicated at the home stations. As one home station provider noted, "There's some value to getting treatment in another environment with the cues of the base removed."

NICoE staff also acknowledged they have the luxury of time that home station sites likely do not: "It's about time. If you have 20 patients and 20 minutes, you can't give them [the] level of care they need. We have that luxury." Some home station providers felt that the differing levels of resources between the NICoE and their home station made it more difficult to manage patient expectations. Although some home station providers were happy with the NICoE's services, they also felt that it should be the NICoE's responsibility to help manage a patient's expectations for follow-on care:

I have to be very careful about telling my patients that you can't expect the rest of the medical care system to operate like that, and it is incumbent upon NICoE to also convey that to them.

Home station providers were particularly vocal about the practical challenges they faced in following the interdisciplinary treatment model of the NICoE. In particular, the single intake session where all providers are present at the initial patient visit was perceived as difficult to implement. While home station providers saw the value in the "tell-your-story" meetings at the NICoE, they also reported that it was difficult to ensure that all providers were present at each meeting.

NICoE sees less than one-third of the patient population we see and has three times the space we have. . . . They do a 'tell-your-story' thing. The team [there] is able to do that. I'm lucky if I can get three bodies in on the 'tell your stories.'

Some providers also did not understand how it was possible to bill for staff when all staff were meeting together with a single patient, at the same time; they wondered how the NICoE accomplished this. They saw full participation in the meetings as a luxury available to the NICoE that might not be possible for the home stations.

Notably, having a "fresh start" to treatment was not always viewed positively among home station providers. Some home station providers argued that the NICoE's emphasis on and confirmation of TBI detracted from the work done at the home stations to get the patient to accept psychological health services for problems co-occurring with or resulting from the TBI. Some providers believed that most concussions would heal naturally and that the underlying cause of the patient's symptoms was often psychological (e.g., related to PTSD). They argued that focusing on the injury was "pathologizing": "Patients are coming back very, very sick." According to these providers, after some patients see their brain scans and are told that they have brain damage, they feel as though they will never get better. After a stay at the NICoE, these providers said, patients tend to focus on the physical damage and dismiss the earlier PTSD diagnosis, which "sets [home station providers] back 20 steps" with their patients and undermines the provider's diagnosis. In the words of one provider, patients come back and say, "See, I told you I had brain damage and not PTSD."

Likewise, home station providers expressed a philosophy of care that seemed to be at odds with the NICoE's perceived mission. Because many of the symptoms of TBI and PTSD overlap, home station providers felt that treating the symptoms of both disorders was sufficient and that the advanced brain scans done at the NICoE were ultimately a distraction from treatment. The home stations seemed to emphasize treatment and focused less on etiology:

They [the NICoE] need more of a treatment model rather than a diagnosis one. NICoE is reviewing the scans with the patients, and this validates for them that it is TBI and that they aren't going to get better. So they don't focus on the PTSD, which is the symptoms.

Finally, rather than serving as a "fresh start" to treatment for all service members who meet the eligibility criteria, some home station providers felt that the NICoE should have a clinical role that primarily serves home stations with few resources. These providers felt that the NICoE should focus on patients without access to the resources of a large military medical hospital or those who must travel extensive distances for more advanced care. In fact, this sense that the NICoE should be reserved for service members who are unable to access care locally often shaped providers' willingness to refer patients to the NICoE. One provider commented, "We have the resources. I don't want them to take a place from someone who needs it," while another said, "Maybe if I were at a facility like [a small treatment facility] that doesn't have many services, I would send [patients] to [the NICoE] all the time."

Conclusion

Although there is some confusion among home station providers and NICoE staff about the mission of the NICoE and its role within the MHS, most agree that the NICoE currently serves a clinical role in providing a "fresh start" to treatment for patients for whom treatment has not yet been effective. However, home station providers are not in agreement about the necessity or the benefits of this service, although most agree that the NICoE fills an important gap in serving patients living far from an MTF or at home stations without adequate resources for treating TBI and psychological health problems. Of note, few of the home station providers and NICoE staff we spoke with mentioned the goal of returning service members to full duty as part of the NICoE's mission. Most providers agreed that a greater understanding of the NICoE's mission and services, as well as a defined relationship between NICoE and home station providers, would be helpful in refining coordination among facilities.

CHAPTER FOUR

Who Is Referred to the NICoE, and How Does the Referral Process Work?

The second aim of this report was to evaluate the process of referral of service members from the home station to the NICoE. The multi-method approach described in Chapter Two provided us with the data to describe the process by which patients are referred to the NICoE for further assessment and individualized treatment. In this chapter, we explore in more detail the NICoE's eligibility criteria, the idiosyncratic criteria used by home station providers to refer service members to the NICoE, the characteristics of service members who are referred, gaps in care at the time of referral, the steps and variability in the referral process, and patient and provider satisfaction with the process.

What Kind of Patients Are Referred to the NICoE for Treatment?

According to referral information on the NICoE website (NICoE, 2014c), service members must meet the following criteria to be eligible for the NICoE:

- Be an active-duty service member from any service branch (including the National Guard and reservists on orders)
- Have a mission-related mild or moderate TBI
- Have comorbid psychological health condition(s)
- Fail to respond to TBI and mental health care offered at the service member's home station
- Have the potential and desire to return to duty.

These criteria were confirmed by NICoE clinicians and administrators during our site visit, with the exception of the potential and desire to return to duty. In practice, NICoE patients include a mix of service members who are expected to return to duty and those who are currently undergoing medical evaluation boards and unlikely to return to full duty. Exclusion criteria include a lack of independence in daily living activities; active, untreated substance use disorders; and any current danger to oneself or others.

Although the NICoE has developed and disseminated materials that describe the eligibility and exclusion criteria for referral to NICoE, home station providers at the sites we visited were not certain about who should be referred to the NICoE, and they reported various strategies for determining whether to make a referral. Several respondents commented that they wished they had more guidance from NICoE about the types of patients to refer. Despite some confusion, many providers reported that they referred patients who had completed treatment at the home base and were not making additional progress in terms of outcomes or functioning. Some providers correctly noted that patients must have both a mild or moderate TBI and a psychological health condition, but others reported that they referred anyone with a mild or moderate TBI. Some providers indicated that they mainly referred service members who were in the process of medical separation from the military because the NICoE's evaluation and treatment recommendations can serve to support the necessary documentation required for this process. Others perceived that service members with a particular need for privacy (e.g., special forces, higher-ranking service members) had increased access to the NICoE. Some providers reported having referred patients to the NICoE to help patients receive necessary treatment outside of the demands of their daily work and home life, with one provider commenting that "Getting care is based on presentation and timing. The concern is operations for [the command]; you work your health care around the operations." Most of the interviewed providers reported that everyone they had referred to the NICoE had been accepted for the program, although some providers whose patients were declined reported frustration with not understanding why certain referrals were not accepted.

In the survey of providers, clinicians reviewed a list of clinical indicators for a NICoE referral and selected all indicators that would lead them to make a referral (Figure 4.1). They also provided their reasons for not referring a patient to the NICoE (Figure 4.2). The most commonly endorsed reasons for referral were that the patient's TBI or psychological health problems were complex and severe (endorsed by 83 percent of respondents) and that the

Figure 4.1
Reasons the Provider Would Refer a Patient to the NICoE

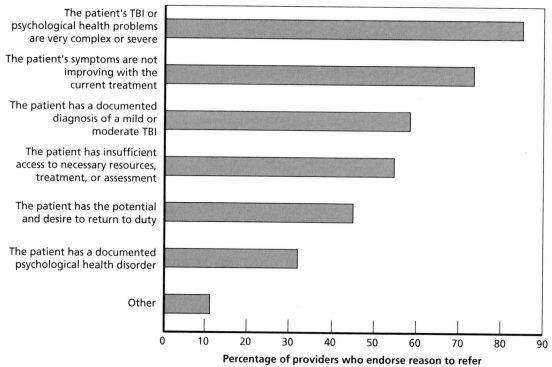

Percentage of providers who endorse reason to refer

Figure 4.2
Reasons the Provider Would Not Refer a Patient to the NICoE

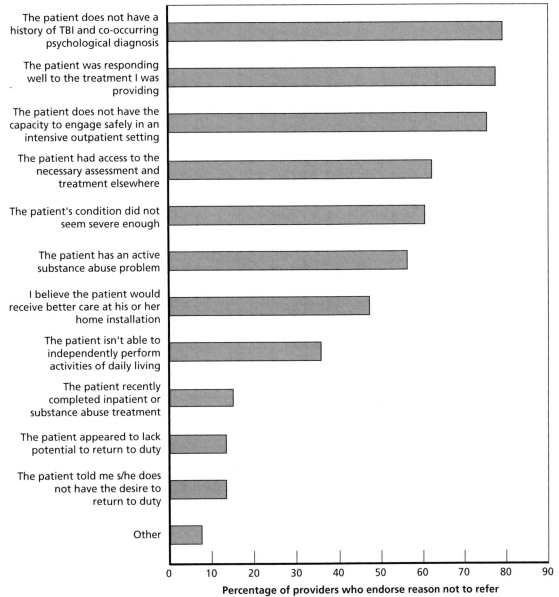

RAND *RR-653-4.2*

patient's symptoms were not improving with the current treatment (endorsed by 72 percent of respondents). These indicators are consistent with the NICoE's eligibility criteria and indicate that three-quarters to four-fifths of providers who have already referred to the NICoE would consider a referral for a patient with these characteristics. The most commonly endorsed reasons for not referring a patient to the NICoE were that the patient did not have TBI and a co-occurring psychological diagnosis, was responding well to the treatment the clinician was providing, or did not have the capacity to engage safely in an outpatient setting (endorsed by approximately three-quarters of respondents).

Not all providers, despite having referred or received at least one NICoE patient, were aware that comorbid mental health conditions were a criterion for acceptance. In addition, although written NICoE materials indicate that NICoE patients must have a desire and capacity to return to active duty, both referring providers and NICoE staff confirmed that many NICoE patients are in the process of leaving the service.

What Problems Are Patients Experiencing at the Time of Referral to the NICoE?

In response to the survey fielded with former NICoE patients, participants retrospectively reported poor functioning in the months preceding the referral to the NICoE. They believed their TBI or psychological health symptoms were moderately (26 percent), severely (50 percent), or extremely (24 percent) impacting their relationships with important others (friends, spouses, children). Occupational functioning was also a concern for the majority of respondents. Three former patients (5 percent) indicated that their TBI or psychological symptoms had only a minimal impact on their work functioning, but most believed their symptoms had a moderate (31 percent), severe (36 percent), or extreme (29 percent) impact on their work functioning.

Participants were asked to identify retrospectively the "most important problem that [they] hoped to address [at the NICoE]." Concentration and memory problems were selected by 29 percent of respondents. Pain was selected by 27 percent of respondents, and psychological or emotional concerns (e.g., posttraumatic stress, depression, anger) were selected by 26 percent of respondents. Few or no participants identified sleep problems (6.5 percent), sensory problems (2 percent), speech and language issues (0 percent), or relationship problems (0 percent) as the primary problem they wished to address at the NICoE. Most respondents indicated that their primary problem was causing severe (55 percent) or extreme (23 percent) distress.

Although survey participants indicated only the most important problem that they had hoped to address at the NICoE, our conversations with former NICoE patients during site visits often revealed complex clinical presentations with symptoms across multiple domains. A typical patient's self-described functioning prior to a NICoE referral can be summarized by the following response:

> Before I went, I was still in pain. My memory was real bad. Headaches. Migraines. It was hard to remember things, to do stuff. I forget what I'm doing half the time. [I was] stagnant. I didn't know what was going to happen with me. I couldn't go back to a regular job.

Referring providers tended to focus less on patient overall functioning at the time of the referral than did patients. Poor functioning and complex presentations are often the norm for specialty providers' caseloads. One provider generalized: "Everybody has short-term memory [problems], daily headaches, and vestibular issues." Instead of overall functioning, providers consistently stated that poor functioning *after* local resources had been exhausted was their referral trigger. The provider quoted above continued: "After they go [through] the 16-week [home station TBI] program and the provider feels they need more testing, especially if there's not much improvement then [they get referred to the NICoE]."

At the Time of Referral to the NICoE, Were There Perceived Gaps in Home Station Care?

During home station site visit interviews, we also asked about the care that patients were and were not able to access prior to referral. There was little consensus in the views of home station providers about gaps in care experienced by patients who were ultimately referred to the NICoE. As described in Chapter Two, the site visit home stations were sampled systematically to ensure representation of sites with TBI and PH resources that ranged from minimal to comprehensive, which likely explains the differing perspectives. Some providers operating within comprehensive TBI clinics felt that there were few gaps in the types of care available, noting that their facility had a state-of-the art assessment and treatment infrastructure. Other providers, at smaller facilities or without a TBI clinic, noted struggling even with basic services, such as access to psychiatric consultations. One of the few common themes across sites was a struggle with heavy caseloads and inadequate staffing. For example, home station providers noted that compared to the NICoE, at their facility "you can't get in as quickly" and the "main stumbling block is having enough providers to do things here." Some providers also noted that complementary and alternative medicine (CAM) treatments, which are available at the NICoE, are not accessible at home stations.

Gaps in care from the patient perspective were assessed through the survey of former NICoE patients and site visit interviews with former NICoE patients. The survey asked respondents to assess their satisfaction with the care they received from their home station prior to attending the NICoE. We note that since these responses were retrospective, respondents' perspective on their pre-NICoE care may have been biased by intervening experiences. Statements about home station care pre-NICoE were rated on a scale from 1 (not at all satisfied) to 5 (completely satisfied). On average, participants were "slightly satisfied" with the care they received for TBI or psychological health conditions at their home station prior to attending the NICoE (mean [M]=2.1, SD=1.2). On average, respondents were less satisfied with the care they received to address their primary concern (e.g., pain, memory problems) (M=1.8, SD=1.0). Respondents reported slight to moderate satisfaction with their relationship with home station providers (M=2.5, SD=1.1) and with their providers' knowledge about TBI and psychological health conditions (M=2.2, SD=1.2). These responses, indicating generally low satisfaction with home station care, may be driven by gaps in the care available at home stations. Alternatively, patients who do not respond to care (an eligibility criterion for NICoE attendance) may be more likely to perceive that care as low quality.

During site visit interviews with former NICoE patients, interviewees' responses echoed the survey conclusions. They described disjointed and noncomprehensive care at their home stations. It was common to hear about home station wait times for first appointments measured in months and time between appointments of four to six weeks. Patients often attributed these problems to staff shortages. One patient acknowledged: "They're absolutely swamped. Definitely they need more people. That's first and foremost." Another patient agreed, noting that they "need more medical officers. [It's a] bottlenecked system so getting care is hard." Other complaints included lack of patient-centered care (e.g., "pretty much someone's cookie cutter idea of how something should be handled. This is what we always do so this is what we are going to do with you") and poor coordination between providers.

What Is the Process to Refer Patients to the NICoE?

Typically, potential NICoE patients are referred by their home station primary care manager (PCM), or primary care provider (PCP), neurologist, or psychiatrist. During the referral process, the home station care provider submits a referral form to the NICoE, usually by fax. This brief form includes 50 items and is two pages in length (NICoE, 2014c) The NICoE uses an eligibility team or "white team" to evaluate the potential patient information and determine whether the patient is eligible for the NICoE's services, and then communicates the decision to the referring provider. Service members who are not accepted to the NICoE receive a recommendation for more appropriate placement or treatment.

During home station site visits, we noted variability with respect to the providers who were responsible for referring patients and the process by which the referral decision was made. At some sites, an interdisciplinary treatment team determined whether patients should be referred to the NICoE. At other sites, patients were referred by individual providers, such as a primary care provider.

In general, the providers with whom we spoke during our site visits reported that the referral process was relatively easy, requiring no more than "just filling out a worksheet and sending it to NICoE." However, one provider commented on the format of the referral application, noting that it "is not user friendly. The Word document is problematic. I have time [to fill it out], but the PCMs don't. An online version where you can click [on a drop-down menu] would be better."

Some providers expressed a desire to have more information from the NICoE about why patients are or are not accepted into the program, to help inform future referrals. One provider commented, "You send the [referral] packet not knowing what [the outcome of the referral will be]. [If we had more information], it would be more effective for us to make a referral with more confidence. Now it's just do and hope."

Our discussions with former NICoE patients during the site visits generally confirmed the impressions of the site providers. That is, patients indicated some variability in who initiated their referral, but they were generally satisfied with the referral process and noted that it proceeded smoothly.

Providers who responded to the online survey had referred an average of 6.6 (SD=11.4) patients to the NICoE, of whom 91 percent were accepted by the NICoE. It was rare for referring providers to make a referral decision without consulting other team members (9 percent did so). The most commonly consulted team members were case managers (62 percent of referring providers consulted with case managers), psychiatrists (49 percent), psychologists (47 percent), and neurologists (32 percent). Fewer of surveyed providers indicated that they consulted with nursing staff (11 percent), occupational therapists (21 percent), physical therapists (23 percent), primary care providers (23 percent), or speech therapists (21 percent) prior to making a NICoE referral.

Most providers who responded to the survey indicated that they were either "very" or "completely satisfied" with the NICoE's referral process (64 percent). However, about one-tenth of respondents indicated that they were "not at all satisfied" with the process (9 percent). Despite general agreement that the referral process was satisfactory, providers nonetheless believed that there were opportunities for improvement. Nearly all respondents (95 percent) "agreed" or "strongly agreed" that including a description of the NICoE eligibility criteria on the referral form would be helpful. The majority of respondents also "agreed" or "strongly agreed" that the process would be improved by use of an electronic referral form (86 percent), a referral link within the electronic medical record (Armed Forces Health Longitudinal Technical Application, or AHLTA) (70 percent), or by shortening the referral processing time (64 percent).

Do Patients Referred to the NICoE Agree to Attend and Complete the Program?

According to survey responses from referring providers, nearly all of the patients whom they referred to the NICoE (and who were accepted) agreed to attend the program (92 percent, $SD=22.2$). During site visit conversations with former NICoE patients, most reported that the decision to attend was an easy one. For example, one former patient explained: "I thought it was a great program when I first heard about it. Everything I heard about it was great. I was definitely interested in going."

According to NICoE staff interviewed at the site visit to the NICoE, nearly all service members who begin treatment at the NICoE complete the four-week assessment and treatment planning period, and only a small number of patients (approximately two to three) had voluntarily left the program early. An additional ten patients (approximately) required transfer to an inpatient or residential care setting due to acute psychiatric or substance abuse issues that could not be safely managed in NICoE's outpatient setting.

Conclusion

The NICoE's eligibility criteria for patient referrals differed somewhat from the criteria used by home station providers. During our site visits, providers who referred patients expressed some uncertainty about the NICoE criteria and why some referrals had been rejected. There was also variability in who initiated the referral process for a given patient, but most providers made their referrals in consultation with team members, including case managers, psychiatrists, and psychologists. The providers surveyed indicated that 92 percent of patients they had referred to the NICoE were accepted.

Surveyed providers' levels of satisfaction with the referral process were moderate, with 64 percent reporting being "very" or "completely" satisfied with the process. Providers indicated that the process could be improved with the inclusion of the NICoE's eligibility criteria on the referral materials, as well as an electronic referral system, a referral link within AHLTA, and a shorter referral processing time.

While providers infrequently cited a lack of access to necessary resources and treatment as a reason for referring a patient to the NICoE, patients in our survey sample articulated low levels of satisfaction with the care received at their home stations. During our site visits, patients also highlighted such concerns as long wait times, disjointed care, and staff shortages, which could indicate that gaps in care are being filled by the NICoE for patients who are referred by their home station providers.

In Chapter Five, we describe the services offered to patients referred to the NICoE and levels of provider, patient, and spouse satisfaction with these services. We also offer insight on the future role of the NICoE's satellite facilities.

NICoE Assessment and Treatment Processes

The third aim of this study was to describe the NICoE assessment and treatment processes, including interactions with the home station during that time. Our survey and site visit interviews included several questions about levels of provider, patient, and spouse satisfaction with the services provided during a patient's stay at the NICoE and the quality of communication with NICoE staff. While opinions of the value of a stay at the NICoE, the facility's care model, and its efforts to involve family members in patient care were positive, some providers noted gaps in the NICoE's communication about patient progress to providers and limited knowledge of the services available at home station facilities. Feedback from home station providers, patients, and spouses offers a general idea of where to focus improvement efforts. Recall that the number of participating spouses was small (*N*=4), and, therefore, the comments summarized below may not capture the full range of spouse experiences.

What Clinical Services Are Offered to NICoE Patients?

A total of 397 patients had received services at the NICoE as of January 2013, shortly before our site visit there. Those patients represented all four service branches and 62 different military installations. Service members from the Army and Marine Corps accounted for the largest proportion of patients treated. The NICoE facility accepts five new patients per week, for a total of 20 patients per month. At the time of our visit to the NICoE, patients had an approximately one-month wait before beginning their care program at the facility.

According to NICoE staff, when a patient begins his or her stay at the NICoE, the first step is to increase the patient's comfort by addressing sleep disturbances and any pain that he or she is experiencing. The second step is to conduct intensive diagnostics to determine how providers can improve or maintain the patient's treatment regimen. The third step is to enhance the patient's ability to be his or her own advocate through education efforts aimed at enhancing self-efficacy and self-advocacy skills. Throughout the process, the patient and his or her family are also educated about the patient's condition(s).

The care provided at the NICoE may incorporate patients' families into the process. During our visit to NICoE headquarters in Bethesda, Maryland, staff indicated that spouses or other family members are welcome to accompany patients for the duration of their stay, but families typically arrive in the third or fourth week or visit for a limited period. While at the NICoE, family members may accompany patients to their appointments and are encouraged to participate in educational activities. NICoE staff stated that their education efforts are primarily intended to help the patient and his or her family better understand the patient's diagnoses, thereby facilitating a successful recovery.

How Satisfied with NICoE Services Are Referring Providers, Patients, and Their Spouses?

Site Provider Perspective

During our site visits and in response to our survey, many referring providers expressed a positive impression of NICoE services. One provider claimed to have "only heard good things about the treatment there" and cited consistently positive experiences with NICoE staff. Providers appreciated the efforts of NICoE staff to educate patients and family members. As one provider noted: "They are very good with education. [Patients] say, 'Now I understand. I get it.'" Some providers also acknowledged the potential benefits of a residential stay, noting that it allows the patient to get away from work and life pressures. The NICoE's integrated approach to behavioral health was emphasized as a positive aspect of the program, and providers were impressed by the fact that "they do everything in 28 days." Consistent with these observations, survey results showed that only 6 percent of referring providers (n=3) were dissatisfied with the NICoE's diagnostic evaluation, while 73 percent (n=36) were "very" or "completely" satisfied.

Consistent with the survey findings, during site visits many home station providers noted that they appreciated the comprehensive, high-quality evaluations and quick turnaround time for services at the NICoE. "They can have the audiologist and the vestibular therapist evaluate the patient simultaneously, and we don't have that," said one provider who also cited sleep studies as a service that home stations struggle to provide but the NICoE easily delivers: "Sixty percent of people with TBI have sleep apnea. Unfortunately, we have to go through TRICARE criteria to get a sleep study. Everyone at NICoE gets a sleep study."

Despite generally positive comments, home station providers also noted a number of concerns. Some providers—particularly those at well-resourced MTFs—did not perceive a significant difference between the types of services offered at the home station and those offered at the NICoE. According to a provider from a large facility, "It's great for the small bases for NICoE to do the diagnosis, but not for us. We can do all of that ourselves." A provider from a smaller facility said that although the traditional TBI services are similar, "[The NICoE is] very wellness-oriented. Many of [the alternative therapies] are enormously helpful."

Other home station providers expressed concern that the NICoE assessment process can appear to question the competency of home station providers by repeating diagnostics that had already been completed. They noted that this practice could contribute to lower levels of patient satisfaction with home station care. Indeed, some providers felt that patients tended to have a lower opinion of the services provided at their home base after receiving additional or different diagnostic information from the NICoE. In the words of one provider, "[It makes it appear as if we are] not competent to do our job if [the patient has] already been through our program and discharged, then the NICoE sends the patient back to us for additional treatment. NICoE always sends them back, and there's always additional care." According to another, "They come back [from a stay at the NICoE] and the results are about the same except for the advanced level tested [referring to the advanced imaging technology used by the NICoE]. The service member says, 'See? They found that something is wrong with my brain and you didn't.'" Others disagreed with the implications of additional assessment work completed at the NICoE, noting that even when assessments differ they can be helpful. One provider noted: "They don't miss a thing. They are really good on picking up on things we've missed."

Some providers described the NICoE's assessments as so comprehensive as to include issues unrelated to patients' TBI and psychological health problems—like a mole or cyst. One provider relayed a conversation with a NICoE patient in which the patient noted: "They were sending me for a cyst and I felt like I was wasting time that I should have been spending on PTSD and TBI evaluations."

Some of those who expressed disappointment with the value of NICoE services said that they had not realized that the NICoE's treatment plan was designed to be implemented by the home station provider. One provider summarized the situation as follows: "The belief system is that NICoE treats people, which is not the case. They provide a wonderful diagnostic assessment and recommendations, but it is the belief [that patients receive treatment]."

Finally, we also heard concerns that the NICoE's focus is limited to TBI, even though TBI and PTSD are often interwoven problems. "They are going after the TBI, without enough addressing of the PTSD. The [mental health] issues are probably not being addressed. You can't separate them out. The problem is that they are additive," said one provider.

Willingness to refer another appropriate patient to the NICoE provides a final proxy of referring provider's satisfaction with NICoE services. In response to a survey item that assessed future referrals, a small number of providers indicated that they would not refer again (*n*=3, 6.3 percent). But the majority of providers indicate that they were "very" or "extremely" likely to refer to the NICoE again (*n*=33, 69 percent), suggesting that nearly seven in ten referring providers believed that NICoE services were helpful.

Patient and Spouse Perspective

There were mixed views among former NICoE patients about the value of a residential stay at the NICoE. Many believed that the NICoE offers a relaxed setting in which the patient can focus on his or her care and mentioned that the NICoE's approach was less medication-focused and more oriented toward CAM and holistic treatment plans. "Those CAM things are definitely helpful. [You] get a break from the normal day and get away from your problems," said one patient. Respondents pointed to such activities as art therapy, yoga, music, Tai Chi, and service dog training as particularly useful in promoting relaxation and general wellness. In general, patients appreciated the opportunity to incorporate CAM activities into their treatment plans, even if they did not enjoy every activity offered: "The guided imagery—I thought that was kind of hokey. The art therapy wasn't my cup of tea; the writing was. They have something for everybody."

Other patients and their spouses believed that some aspects of the environment at the NICoE were not suited to the needs of those with anxiety symptoms and sleep problems. For example, one patient reported that he or she was hesitant to speak freely among higher-ranking personnel. Others thought that being in an unfamiliar environment had exacerbated preexisting sleep problems: "You have this one room, it destroys your sleep hygiene. . . . [My] sleep got worse while I was up there."

Despite these concerns, patients and their spouses who participated in our survey and interviews felt that the NICoE's value was in the personal attention given to patients by a team of providers, the ability to develop integrated and individualized treatment plans that take into account multiple problems, and the flexibility of the treatment options. "If you have a lot of issues, that's definitely the place to go," said one patient. A spouse highlighted the advantages of the NICoE's team-based approach to intake by saying that the patient "liked not having to tell the story to ten different people," adding that there is a risk of leaving out important details when meeting with multiple providers individually, particularly in cases in which patients suffer from memory impairment. We heard from other patients and their spouses that NICoE staff related well to patients and were "incredibly accommodating," supported "whatever works for the individual," and were "quick to make adjustments" if the patient was not satisfied with aspects of the treatment plan or required additional support. According to one patient,

> The whole thing was pretty interactive the whole way through: "This is what we have in mind and this is what we're going to stick with. Let's see how it works, then we'll adjust." And if you felt you needed to adjust or deviate, if you had good cause, they were very receptive on that. They absolutely learned and implemented on the fly. They were pretty clear that it wasn't a cookie-cutter treatment plan.

Patients and their spouses frequently mentioned the value of the NICoE's education services, adding that the staff provided a clear explanation of the patient's diagnosis. NICoE staff "helped explain a lot of the things that were going on with me, gave me understanding. They teach you how to be your own advocate, they give the diagnosis, they tell you what the symptoms are of TBIs," said one patient, who described attending classes on the topic. According to another, the staff "understood where we were coming from. We weren't looked at like we were . . . making stuff up or damaged goods. . . . It was very supportive."

Many respondents appreciated the comprehensiveness and efficiency of the evaluations and treatment recommendations, noting that NICoE staff addressed everything from sleep and headache problems to minor complaints. According to one respondent, "The attitude of [NICoE] providers is to take care of you and figure out what's wrong. They want to look at every inch of your body to figure out what's going on." Like home station providers, patients and their spouses were impressed by the speed with which NICoE staff conducted diagnostic tests and developed treatment plans. One patient contrasted the quick turnaround time for diagnostic services with that for the care received at home, adding, "Everything was fast-paced, but it was well thought out." Others liked the idea of "knocking out six months of appointments in four weeks."

At the NICoE, patients are assessed using a variety of advanced neuroimaging technologies, such as magnetic resonance imaging (MRI) and magneto encephalography (MEG). The results of the neuroimaging assessments are shared with the patient and sometimes are suggestive of brain lesions, which can be viewed as physical evidence of the TBI. Patients we spoke with at site visits had mixed views upon seeing their neuroimaging results, with some questioning their value for TBI diagnoses. For example, one patient's neuroimaging results did not show any lesions, leading the patient to question the reason for other physical symptoms indicating TBI, such as recurring headaches. Another patient whose scan revealed many lesions felt that the NICoE's diagnosis merely confirmed what the patient already knew—and that a stay at the NICoE was an unnecessary investment of time and money. Other patients saw substantial value in being able to see visual evidence of their injuries. "All the different MRIs they did, they found a lot more stuff wrong with my back. They were able to physically show me my TBI," said one patient. The comments and suggestions provided by former NICoE patients during site visits were generally consistent with the online survey of former NICoE patients. According to survey results, overall satisfaction with the care received at the NICoE was high; the vast majority of former patients indicated that they were "very" or "completely" satisfied with their care at the NICoE (93.5 percent). Satisfaction with care specific to their "major concern" (e.g., pain, psychological concerns) was also high (88.7 percent of respondents were "very" or "completely" satisfied). Nearly all former NICoE patients who completed the survey indicated that they were "very" or "completely" satisfied with their therapeutic relationship with their NICoE providers (96.8 percent) and were similarly satisfied with their providers' knowledge of TBI and/or psychological health concerns (98.8 percent).

Table 5.1 summarizes former patients' preferences regarding the degree of focus on various components of care for TBI and psychological health concerns. In general, patients believed that either the amount of assessment or treatment in various domains was "just right" or they would have preferred to receive more of it. It was less common for former patients to indicate that they would have liked to receive less of a given assessment or treatment approach.

Overall, home station providers and patients and their spouses found that the comprehensive assessments and individual attention provided by the NICoE were useful for patients' treatment and general well-being. Both groups expressed some concerns about the treatment suggestions and the utility of a second round of diagnostic testing. Some providers' reservations about referring patients to the NICoE were tied to an implication of subpar treatment or capability at patients' home stations. This concern may indicate a need for more outreach to home station providers to clarify their role, and the NICoE's intent to augment rather than serve as a substitute for the services provided on base.

Table 5.1
Percentage of Former NICoE Patients Who Would Have Preferred More or Fewer NICoE Assessment and Treatment Services

Please rate the extent to which you would have preferred more or less of each aspect of NICoE services	1 Shorter, Fewer, or Less	2	3 Just Right	4	5 Longer or More
Length of stay at the NICoE	1.7	0	31.7	10.0	56.7
Number of assessments/tests	0	1.7	56.7	13.3	28.3
Number of individual counseling sessions	1.7	3.3	38.3	20.0	36.7
Number of group counseling sessions	17.2	12.1	44.8	10.3	15.5
Amount of computer/simulation training	16.3	4.1	42.9	14.3	22.4
Amount of complementary and alternative medicine (like acupuncture or yoga)	0	5.1	15.3	23.7	55.9
Amount of opportunities to build my skills to manage my TBI	0	0	33.3	25.0	41.7
Number of physical exams by doctors	0	0	80.0	8.3	11.7

How Satisfied Are Providers, Patients, and Spouses with Communication During Care at the NICoE?

Interdisciplinary Meetings Within the NICoE

During a patient's stay at the NICoE, he or she interacts with an interdisciplinary team of providers responsible for different components of the assessment and treatment plan. The team meets with a patient upon his or her arrival at the NICoE, which helps ensure that the patient is not required to restate the same information multiple times to many different providers. The intake appointment also gives the team a starting point to collaborate and develop an individualized plan for the patient's care. "When I got to the NICoE, I explained to them what treatments I was already getting. Everyone was well in the loop about what was going on," said one patient.

Communication Between the NICoE and Referring Providers

Providers' satisfaction with the degree of communication with NICoE during a patient's stay was mixed. In response to the online survey of referring providers, most respondents indicated that they were "very" or "completely" satisfied with the frequency (73.4 percent) and quality (75.6 percent) of their communication with the NICoE. However, there was a substantial minority that was "not at all satisfied" with the frequency (13.3 percent) and quality (11.1 percent) of their communication with the NICoE. Moreover, three-quarters (75 percent) of respondents believed that the NICoE's recommendations would be improved by "increased communication between providers at the NICoE and the home station."

Some clinic administrators at home station treatment facilities reported regular communication between the NICoE and their sites: "We consult with them on an informal basis pretty regularly. NICoE people have come here at least twice and we've sent some of our staff up there." However, there appears to be an opportunity for greater or more targeted communication between NICoE staff and referring providers. For example, some providers indicated that it would be helpful for the NICoE to provide ongoing, in-person briefings to site staff and for the NICoE to maintain records of the services available at each home station, along with key points of contact to facilitate communication and updates. According to one provider, it had been "years since [the] first brief. I can't think of anyone that's been back since." Some providers noted that the rapid rotation of clinicians at home station facilities, given the military deployment cycle and change of stations, makes it more challenging to ensure that new providers are informed of the services offered at the NICoE.

Citing concerns about duplication of services, referring providers suggested that a better mutual understanding of the services available at the patient's home station and at the NICoE would prevent redundancy of care and would help guide decisions about which patients to refer to the NICoE. One provider suggested, "Maybe if we had a list of their services and they had a list of our services, we could maybe not overlap as much, and we could just utilize them for the resources they have that we don't and vice versa." Another stated, "We understand . . . the way things work here. They should listen to our guidance here."

Some providers confirmed that they communicated with NICoE staff on a regular basis while their referred patients were in residence at the NICoE. Their primary point of contact was the patient's NICoE case manager, with whom providers discussed patients' progress and treatment plans. Many providers found NICoE staff both accessible and responsive, and they were satisfied with the updates provided. "It's been pretty smooth. I was amazed at how accessible they were," said one provider, adding that NICoE staff were "pretty good about calling you back and keeping you updated." However, other providers indicated that they had little or no communication with the NICoE and believed that this was an area for improvement. One provider concluded, "They probably aren't reading our notes. There's the lack of communication there." Another cited time constraints as interfering with good communication:

> I don't have time to sit in an hour discharge meeting. I don't get calls. Upfront, I get the email response from admissions saying they are going to review the packet and an email stating [the patient has] been accepted, and then we get an email saying they are preparing for discharge and want to discuss, but by then as far as medication management things are concerned, they've already been done.

It is possible that NICoE case managers were communicating with home station case managers instead of home station providers. One case manager reported having "tons of communication with one of the case managers at NICoE" before, during, and after the patient's stay. Another stated that communication was more "informal" but routine between NICoE and home station case managers.

In some cases, specialty providers at home stations were not even aware that their patients had been to the NICoE (perhaps because NICoE staff typically communicate with the referring provider or case managers). "We never know anyone is up there until they are back here. [It] would be helpful to have a heads-up on the front end," said one provider. These providers believed that adversarial relationships could be prevented by discussing patients' status and treatment history with all providers involved with their care:

> There should be more of a hand-off in both directions [with providers] working more closely together so it's not the A-team and B-team and then the patient. It was an adversarial relationship before. Like, they're going [to the NICoE] because [our facility] had failed them.

In line with the previous comment, some home station providers described NICoE staff as dismissive and felt subordinated in interactions about their patients' evaluation and treatment. According to one such provider, the relationship between the NICoE and home stations "doesn't feel collaborative. . . . [It] feels like they're saying, 'We're better than you.'" Another agreed: "We feel incredibly dismissed. No one has requested any information from us. They have to acknowledge the concerns that we have." One provider relayed an incident in which he or she had prescribed a medication two weeks before the patient's stay at the NICoE. According to the provider, the patient "came back with a different medication. I told them over and over that we had discussed this. They didn't listen to me." It is notable that even after negative experiences, some providers continued to be responsive to increased communication with the NICoE. For example, one provider reported that:

> Recently, their physicians up there called me. I loved that. I would like that to increase, including during the patient's stay at the NICoE, especially since one of their goals is to get these guys back to active duty. To let us know about their thought processes allows us to get a better understanding.

Communication Between the NICoE and Patients and Their Spouses

The NICoE places a high value on involving family members in a patient's care, but family members reported a range of experiences at the NICoE. Some spouses felt more involved at the NICoE than at the patient's home station facility and found the education provided to them to be both helpful and thorough. Others had the impression that spouses were "an afterthought" in the NICoE's approach to care—specifically, it was not clear what role they played in the process or how that role was integrated with the patient's stay at the NICoE. Patients and spouses who found NICoE staff to be informative and helpful gave several examples of positive experiences, describing how education offered to both partners left them feeling better informed: "We feel more educated, like we have a better way forward after NICoE." Others noted practical advantages of spouses being present at meetings with providers. For example, one patient noted: "[My spouse] was able to fill in memory gaps. She liked to participate. She's upset that she was never part of the process, except at NICoE."

Some patients and spouses mentioned that it would be helpful to have more information about what to expect prior to admission to the NICoE: "It would be helpful if NICoE provided a brochure, video or other info for service members and their spouses so they know what to expect." A patient expressed frustration about not receiving a thorough overview of the activities available at the NICoE prior to arriving:

> They have something for everybody, but you don't know what you don't know. They need to give you the round robin quicker. At the end of each week—fill this out on what you want to do for the next week. But you don't know what these things are.

Patients' and spouses' feedback regarding their communication with the NICoE about the patients' treatment plan was generally positive, citing "clear-cut recommendations" and a better understanding of "what the way forward would look like." They also appreciated the NICoE's efforts to "frame the problems so that they could be understood." Few interviewees reported difficulty getting "straight answers" to questions.

Conclusion

With a few exceptions (e.g., integrated education for families and complementary and alternative treatment approaches), many providers did not perceive a significant difference between the types of services offered at the home station and those offered at the NICoE. Some providers felt that patients tended to have a lower opinion of the services provided at their home base after receiving additional or different diagnostic information from the NICoE. In general, however, providers highlighted the individual attention that NICoE staff are able to provide to patients and their families and rated patients' satisfaction with their stay at the NICoE as overwhelmingly positive.

NICoE case managers were seen as a natural point of contact for home station providers and case managers; however, providers noted gaps in the way information is shared, such as whether specialty providers are included in communications. Some providers also felt subordinate or dismissed by NICoE staff when discussing patients' care. Many in this group indicated that additional communication from the NICoE, including in-person sessions with home station providers, would improve mutual understanding of the services provided at each facility.

The NICoE places a significant emphasis on education and the opportunity for family members to be informed and involved in a patient's care. Patients and their spouses had generally positive impressions of the NICoE's efforts. We heard some suggestions from patients and their spouses that communication could be improved prior to patients' admission to the NICoE, with more information about what to expect during the stay and a more clearly defined role for family members who accompany patients. Overall, patients and their spouses who participated in our interviews believed that the NICoE's value was in the personal attention provided to patients by a team of providers, the ability to develop integrated and individualized treatment plans that take into account multiple problems, and the flexibility of the treatment options provided.

In Chapter Six, we take a closer look at the NICoE's discharge process and provider, patient, and spouse perspectives on the transition from a stay at the NICoE to patients' regular care environments.

Transitioning from the NICoE to the Home Station

The fourth aim of this study was to evaluate the patient's process of transitioning back to the home station and home station providers' implementation of the NICoE recommendations. Following complete and comprehensive evaluations of all levels of patient functioning, NICoE staff develop individualized recommendations for follow-up care. The NICoE's diagnostic findings and recommendations are described in a discharge summary intended to direct the treatment the patient will receive when he or she returns to the home station. This chapter provides a description of the NICoE's discharge process, the discharge summary and recommendations, the process of transitioning from the NICoE back to the home station, and the extent to which recommended services are implemented at home stations. We end this chapter by describing patients' and providers' views about the facilitators and barriers to implementing the NICoE's recommendations.

The NICoE Discharge Planning Process

During our visit to the NICoE, we learned that the discharge planning process requires collaboration between the interdisciplinary team of NICoE providers and case managers, the home station providers and case manager, and the patient and his or her family. One NICoE staff person said discharge planning "can be challenging, depending on where they are heading back to." For instance, they noted some service members return to communities and home stations with many resources available or have involved case managers to coordinate care, while others do not. They reported that NICoE specialists provide input on the treatment plan to the NICoE primary care provider, who consolidates the treatment recommendations and finalizes them with feedback from the patient. At the end of the patient's stay at the NICoE, there is a discharge planning teleconference where representatives from the NICoE treatment team meet with the patient and his or her home station provider(s) to review and discuss the treatment plan. One NICoE staff member noted, "We ask the service member who they'd like to have on the [discharge planning] call." When asked about the interaction between the home station and NICoE providers on the call, a NICoE staff member said home station providers "listen, then ask questions. It is normally the [home station] behavioral health provider [who is on the call] if they are the referring provider. Sometimes there is interaction between the service member and [home station] case manager, where the case manager will say 'come see me,' or arrange the follow-up on the phone."

When asked about their involvement with the NICoE discharge planning process, most former NICoE patients reported that they played an active role in finalizing the treatment plan and recommendations. For example, one individual said patients "have veto power on what-ever they put in there." Another reported,

> I was pretty involved. They had a sit down with me and went over the entire thing. My discharge summaries, we went over all that. First they gave me a copy; I went over it and noted where things needed to be changed or added. They sat down with me and did a tele-conference and talked about the changes and all that stuff.

Many, but not all, of the providers we spoke with at site visits had participated in a patient's discharge meeting. Providers had positive things to say about these opportunities to discuss the NICoE's recommendations and treatment plan. One said, "The multidisciplinary conference call at the end was great" and another provider described the meetings as "awe-some." The primary complaint about these meetings came from providers who had encoun-tered scheduling conflicts that prevented them from attending. One provider suggested more scheduling flexibility and advance notice of the meeting: "There is no flexibility on when the discharge meeting is going to be held so it's almost impossible for other providers to participate. They get a couple days' notice." Overall, providers seemed interested in participating in the NICoE discharge planning process if such logistical barriers could be overcome.

The NICoE Discharge Summary and Recommendations

The survey of former NICoE patients assessed patient perspectives of the NICoE discharge summary. Respondents indicated what the NICoE had recommended they do to continue addressing their primary complaint following discharge. Over half of patients reported that the NICoE had recommended they engage in memory strengthening tasks, engage in alternative therapies, and talk with a psychologist or therapist (see Figure 6.1). Other common recommen-dations were that the patient engage in self-care and see a pain specialist, a physical therapist, or a primary care provider regularly. In interviews with former NICoE patients during site visits, patients made similar observations that both traditional and complementary approaches to TBI and psychological health conditions had been recommended by the NICoE. One patient quickly summarized that "NICoE recommended meds, Botox, therapy, and a case manager." Another listed a plan for swimming therapy, continued work with a social worker, and follow-up appointments with speech and language, neurology, and behavioral health providers.

The NICoE staff we met with agreed that the discharge summary is very important. One NICoE staff member said, "The culmination of [the patient's] time at NICoE is a dis-charge document—one document that is seamless. We all sign it collectively. It says about the NICoE, 'this is one visit.'" According to another, "The discharge summary is a roadmap. It is the diagnosis. This is the way forward. If I'm in the office [at the home station], I don't even know where to begin. The hope is that if you have this as a roadmap, we've got some of the big diagnostic questions nailed down."

However, NICoE staff also agreed that it is challenging to write the discharge summary, because it must consolidate findings from diverse disciplines into a coherent summary and set of recommendations that can be implemented at the home station. "Part of the challenge is that there are so many moving pieces. Sometimes a challenge is how specific to be in our recommendations given the resources back home. We try to anticipate their future through

Figure 6.1
The NICoE Recommendations to Continue Addressing Primary Complaint Following Discharge

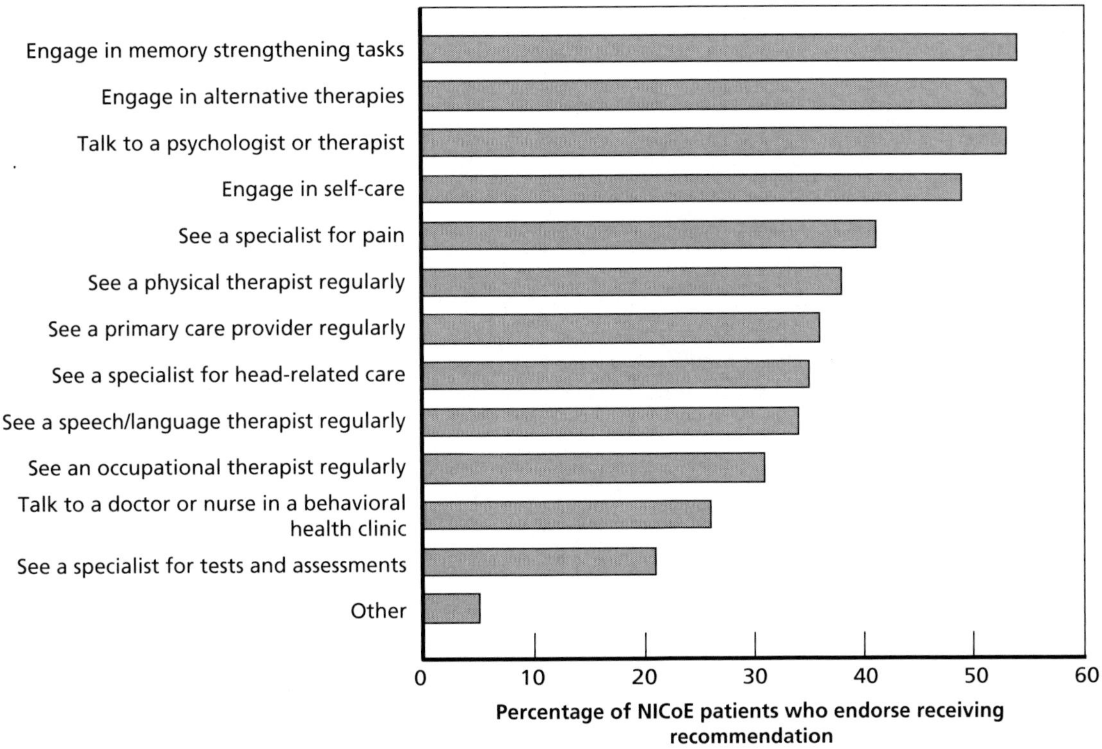

NOTE: Percentages adjusted to exclude missing data.

the Services' medical systems and the VA. We try to say 'this is what we found, and this is what we think will continue the trajectory.'" In addition to adapting the summary based on the patient's access to medical resources, NICoE staff noted other difficulties, such as tailoring the report to be appropriate and useful for different audiences. One explained, "Primary Care Managers [PCMs] at the NICoE are the translators of the discharge summary. They are writing to both the providers and the patients. There are multiple audiences for the document." The length of the document was also noted as a challenge: "They are too cumbersome to put together. PCMs spend hours on each patient's discharge summary. There's just so much finalizing they have to do. . . . There has been controversy over the length of the 20-page discharge summary." Another said a key area where the NICoE could improve would be "streamlining the discharge summaries."

The former NICoE patients and spouses we spoke with generally held positive views on the discharge summary and recommendations. They noted that because they had been involved in discharge planning at the NICoE, their feedback had been incorporated into the recommendations. One former patient called the discharge summary the "golden document," noting it made a difference in the TBI care he or she received after leaving the NICoE. Another former NICoE patient cited the discharge summary's coverage of TBI and PTSD as "gold in my book," but added that some components of the summary are less useful. The patient said, "Some of this is piddly. You've got a military medical document that says you have a hangnail."

There was variation in the extent to which patients believed their home station care providers supported the NICoE's recommendations. One former NICoE patient indicated that his provider "agreed with everything" and another believed that the NICoE's recommendations were consistent with his provider's approach (e.g., "What had been recommended in the treatment plan was kind of what we were doing anyway. They concurred that we were on the right track."). Others believed that their providers did not value or disagreed with the NICoE recommendations (e.g., "Nothing happens when you get back. The folks here say that NICoE blows things way out of proportion.").

Providers generally agreed that "the discharge summary is very thorough," with some referring to the discharge summary as "the 20-page document." Many providers praised the NICoE discharge summary for its comprehensiveness and interdisciplinary coverage. For instance, one said, "it's nice how they summarize everything on there. All the different disciplines in one document." One provider stated that he or she was "pleasantly surprised by the in-depth, head to toe evaluation. It clearly laid out the recommendations. You just need to pick them up and do it. Nothing seemed confusing, and all rationale made sense." On the other hand, some providers believed that the NICoE assessment was too thorough, and in some cases, produced recommendations that were not likely to improve functioning.

> The recommendation of low-t [testosterone] for 31-year-old male is absurd because if you turn enough rocks over you'll find something. First do no harm. Why? What are you looking for? They do every study. I have a list of all the labs they do. It's ridiculous. This would never occur anywhere else on the planet, and then the recommendation is take a multivitamin."

Many providers suggested that shorter summaries would be easier to navigate. A few providers recommended that the discharge summary have a "bottom line up-front" and that it be "broken up so that it is easily readable." One provider explained, "Everything is well-worded, but it's just a lot to read. It's hugely verbose. At some point an editor would be great. They could make bullet points, and shorten it up. The document is useful for the service member to have, but should be more concise regarding follow-up care." Another specifically suggested minimizing the description of patient history if it is already documented elsewhere: "[the discharge summary] describes the history of multiple TBIs, but we already knew that when he went up there. A lot is repetitive with the history." Of note, while many providers at the site visits complained about the length of the discharge summary, only 25 percent of provider survey respondents agreed that shortening its length would improve the quality of the NICoE's recommendations. This suggests that while length can be cumbersome, it does not always impact the perceived quality of the treatment plan.

A few providers viewed the NICoE discharge summaries as confusing. For example, one provider said the document was "almost a mixture of provider notes and patient pages. I can't decide whether the discharge summaries are notes for providers or for the patients, so they are kind of condescending and not appropriate for the physician audience." Another agreed, describing the summaries as "a little offensive, especially when we send [the patient to the NICoE] after they've received care here already. Sometimes the recommendations are what we've already done. Did [the NICoE] read our notes?"

Indeed, while some providers found the recommendations helpful, appropriate, and feasible (e.g., "We do learn things from their recommendations, helps to tweak our treatment plan"), many felt that the recommendations were duplicative of the assessment or services they had already provided to the patient. They recommended that the author of the NICoE discharge summary "make it evident that you've read the person's chart before NICoE, and that the person's previous chart was incorporated into the treatment plan." Some also noted their reluctance to implement certain "controversial" recommendations, (e.g., "treatment for low-t [testosterone]"). Some recounted cases where a provider was not able or willing to administer the treatment the NICoE recommended for the patient, leading to tension between the patient and provider. One provider explained, "The patient has these expectations created, and then 'sorry we don't agree with your opinion' and I have to mediate."

The Transition from the NICoE Back to the Home Station

During site visit interviews with former NICoE patients and their spouses, we asked about the transition from the NICoE back to their home station. Some had experienced smooth transitions. For example, one patient appreciated the collaboration between the NICoE and home station providers and noted that the providers "pretty much set up what I needed to do and what would benefit me back home." Another former NICoE patient said, "before I came home, there was already the understanding that I would be coming [to the TBI clinic]. They worked all that out. I think they communicated that back pretty well." One patient mentioned that "consults were put in from NICoE to help get in the door fast, then there was a VTC [video teleconference] follow-up with home station providers."

However, many former NICoE patients and spouses encountered challenges transitioning back to care at the home station ("the discharge didn't seem as smooth as it could have been"). One specific issue reported was that home station providers seemed unaware of or unable to access the NICoE's discharge summary. One patient expressed frustration that although his or her case manager "supposedly gave [the NICoE discharge summary] to everybody, but somehow nobody knew about it. It never seemed to get into the hands of the people I was seeing." Another said his home station providers "didn't even look at the discharge summary." Patients said the transition was particularly difficult when treatments or services the NICoE recommended were unavailable at or near the home station. To address this issue, several patients recommended better preparation and communication between the two sets of providers and the patient. One suggested that "future NICoE patients get appointments going before they leave the NICoE," and another said it would be helpful if "there could be a list of area providers that take TRICARE and cover the things we learned at NICoE." It was recommended that patients leaving the NICoE "know who and where you're going for the acupuncture or biofeedback, and it's already set up. Your doctor should be answering."

Of the 54 providers who responded to the web-based survey, 44 (81.5 percent) said they had read a NICoE discharge summary. Those reporting they saw at least one patient after discharge from the NICoE on the provider survey ($n=37$, 1 missing response) indicated they had evaluated or treated a mean of 9.1 patients ($SD=14.1$) after return from the NICoE. Providers' responses regarding their preferred method for accessing the NICoE discharge summary are shown below in Figure 6.2 While nearly half of providers ($n=26$, 48 percent) liked being able to view the summary in the patient's medical record, most respondents said they would also like some form of direct communication with the NICoE, by receiving the discharge summary from the NICoE directly ($n=36$, 67 percent) or discussing it on the telephone ($n=11$,

Figure 6.2
Provider Survey Respondents' Preferences for Accessing the NICoE Discharge Summary

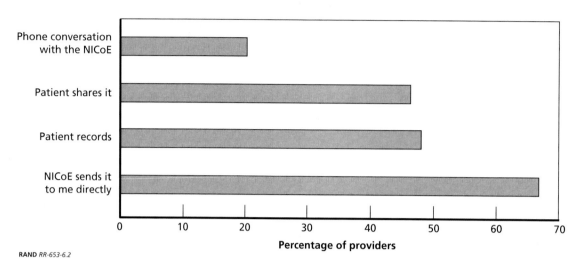

RAND *RR-653-6.2*

NOTE: Respondents could check all options that applied.

20 percent). Having a patient share the summary was desired by nearly half (*n*=25, 46 percent) of providers as well.

Similar to the range of responses we heard from patients, providers described both positive and negative experiences with the transition of patients from the NICoE to the home station. Many providers believed the transition process was working well: "When [the patient] got back to [the home station], he had all his appointments set up. We all knew what to expect when he came home." One provider was pleased that "they don't recommend something we can't use, and if they know we don't have something, they recommend that the soldier get that service somewhere else. They either send the referral themselves for any unavailable services, or they ask us to do it."

On the other hand, several providers highlighted challenges with the transition from the NICoE to the home station and areas for improvement. For instance, some noted that communication about the patient goes from the NICoE to the referring provider but may never reach the patient's other providers. One suggested the NICoE "consider all treating providers on the back end." Another provider specifically suggested that there be a "multidisciplinary team meeting when [the patient] comes back to review the plan with the patient." In addition, a few providers recommended that the NICoE interact and collaborate more with providers at home stations, especially when it is unclear whether a NICoE-recommended treatment is available: "You should have an idea of what's available [at the home station] and work with the folks who are going to implement it. . . . You shouldn't just give the information, but also train the people. . . . They need to make sure that someone at the home base can do [the treatment]."

The Implementation of the NICoE Recommendations at the Home Station

On the provider survey, most home station providers who had referred a patient to the NICoE indicated that the NICoE's recommendations had influenced the treatment they provided to the patient. According to survey responses, 59 percent of referring providers indicated that the treatment they provided to their patient post-NICoE was "very much" or "extremely" influenced by NICoE treatment recommendations. Only a small proportion of providers (5 percent) indicated that the patient's treatment had "not at all" been influenced by NICoE treatment recommendations.

Interviews with home station providers during site visits generally supported this finding. Most providers indicated that all or nearly all of the NICoE's treatment recommendations had been implemented.

> There isn't much that we can't do when they come back. Their recommendations are always doable.

> Discharge summaries are encyclopedic, very thorough. Sometimes we just can't offer vision therapy. It's hard to offer some of the things they recommend, but we do the best we can, and if we can't offer it, at least the patient has it documented.

As described earlier, some providers reported that the NICoE recommendations are not always implemented, sometimes because the provider believes the recommendation had already been tried in the past and other times because administrative hurdles made implementation difficult.

> With the recommendations, I follow orders and also use my clinical judgment. I've talked to the clinic manager, and I'll say we've maximized his potential. I have done that [already].

> We have capability to meet recommendations, but is it hard? Do we have to jump through hoops? Does it always happen? No.

During interviews with NICoE staff and administrators, it appeared that the current system returns little information to the NICoE about what recommendations are or are not implemented by home station providers. One NICoE provider acknowledged, "We don't really know what happens when they go home. We only know if the patient or provider contacts us. It's like a black box." Other NICoE staff worried about this information void and the possibility that they might be recommending care that the patient would not be able to access:

> Is it harmful to tease them here with things they can't get back home? What's the ethical component to that? Give them pain relief, but does it make them more upset in the long run? How can we track progress longitudinally? We don't know what's making them feel better.

According to information we received during a site visit to the NICoE headquarters, the NICoE has partnered with the DVBIC Care Coordination Program to begin to longitudinally track NICoE patients after discharge. It is possible that data from follow-up interviews with NICoE patients about the care received will improve NICoE staff members' understanding of home station resources and the likelihood of recommendations being implemented, which may in turn help providers to tailor discharge recommendations to the patient resources at their home stations.

Our survey of former NICoE patients provided a snapshot of the services patients report receiving at their home stations. About one-half of former NICoE patients indicated that they receive their current care at an MTF (53 percent); one-fifth received care from a VA facility (20 percent); one-fifth from civilian providers (22 percent), and a small number indicated that they received care elsewhere (5 percent). Patients reported seeing a variety of providers for care. Slightly more than one-half of patients saw a primary care physician; about one-half saw a psychiatrist, and one-half saw a neurologist (see Figure 6.3). Patients identified a variety of providers as their key provider,[1] but the most common key providers were neurologists (22 percent), therapists or counselors (18 percent), and psychiatrists (13 percent). Over half of former NICoE patients met with their key provider regularly, that is, at least weekly (25 percent) or monthly (32 percent). Some patients met with their key providers only a few times a year (25 percent), one time only (13 percent), or never (5 percent). Half of former NICoE patients had long-term treatment relationships with their key providers (1–3 years; 49 percent); one-quarter had been seeing their providers for six to 12 months (26 percent), and one-quarter had just begun seeing their providers (0–6 months, 26 percent).

Figure 6.3
Provider Types Serving Former NICoE Patients and Identified Key Providers

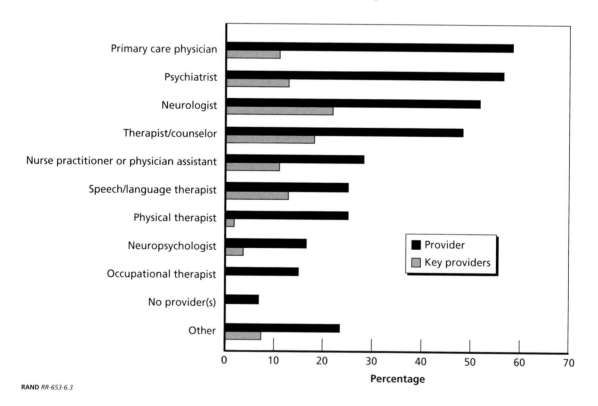

NOTE: Percentages adjusted to exclude missing data.

---

[1]   The patient survey defined a key provider as the provider "who knows the most about the treatment you receive for TBI and/or psychological health conditions."

Survey respondents were asked to describe how informed their key provider was about the recommendations they received from the NICoE. The response scale ranged from 1 (not at all informed) to 5 (completely informed). The average response on the scale was 3.5 (*SD*=1.40). Over half of all patients indicated that they thought that their key provider was either "very informed" (20 percent) or "completely informed" (35 percent).

Former NICoE patients interviewed during site visits had a wide range of experiences with care after they returned to their home stations. Some patients felt that their services abruptly stopped when they returned home, some continued receiving traditional services like primary care or neurology but had difficulty accessing complementary and alternative medicine services, while others were able to easily access all the services recommended by the NICoE. For example:

> I came back here and they told me that they didn't think that the NICoE stuff was right or going to be implemented. I got blowback from the folks here. Where the ball was dropped was with the follow-through when I came back.

> Whenever I got home, TRICARE said there's no way we're going to pay for you to get Botox. You're crazy. My case manager tried to get it set up. TRICARE shot it down.

> I've had no problems with the follow up care, said we can do everything and it won't be an issue.

Facilitators and Barriers to Implementing NICoE Recommendations

On both the NICoE patient and referring provider surveys, participants responded to a series of questions about the facilitators and barriers to implementing NICoE recommendations. Items were phrased differently to correspond to the perspective of each type of respondent, but otherwise reflected the same potential barrier or facilitator.[2] Respondents indicated their level of agreement with each item on a scale from 1 (strongly disagree) to 5 (strongly agree). For ease of interpretation, endorsement is described as the proportion of respondents who indicated that they agreed or strongly agreed with each item.

Facilitators to Implementing NICoE Recommendations

Among NICoE patients, the most commonly endorsed facilitators to getting the care recommended by the NICoE were that the patient wanted the recommended care (97 percent) and believed that the care would help to reduce his or her symptoms (90 percent). Among referring providers, the most commonly endorsed facilitators mimicked those endorsed by patients, that is, when the provider perceived the patient as wanting the recommended care (98 percent) and believing that the care would help to reduce his or her symptoms (98 percent). There were also

---

[2]   For example, one item on the patient survey read, "My doctor makes it mandatory for me to receive the recommended treatment," while the corresponding item on the provider survey read, "I make it mandatory for him or her to receive the treatment."

discrepancies in the frequency with which patients and providers endorsed certain facilitators. For example, 71 percent of providers thought that accessibility of the recommended treatment in the patient's area was a facilitator, while only 38 percent of patients agreed. Similarly a large majority of providers agreed that their belief in the recommended treatment (87 percent) and the commander's support for the service member getting the treatment (89 percent) were facilitators. However, only 60 percent and 55 percent of patients, respectively, thought that these were facilitators to obtaining the care recommended by the NICoE. See Table 6.1 for complete responses from patients and referring providers.

During interviews with former NICoE patients, patients identified improved communication and advocacy skills (gained during the NICoE stay) as a facilitator to obtaining NICoE recommended care. One patient indicated that his or her care had been improved by "standing up for myself and being involved with care." Similarly, another patient discussed improved capacity to communicate with his providers as a facilitator to obtaining needed services:

> Being able to better explain symptoms better, some of that I knew about my spine injury, I was able to go back to my neurosurgeon and explain what still needed to be fixed. Made it easier to talk to treatment providers.

This was consistent with comments from NICoE staff who explicitly noted working with patients to improve their self-advocacy skills. For example, one NICoE provider told us, "We try to reinforce that they should be their own advocate. Just because they've had a bad session, they should try again, and can try another provider."

Barriers to Implementing NICoE Recommendations

Relative to the facilitator items, barriers to care were endorsed by a smaller proportion of patients and providers. Among former NICoE patients, the most commonly endorsed bar-

Table 6.1
Patient- and Home Station Provider-Identified Facilitators to Receiving NICoE Recommended Care

Facilitators to Care	Percent Endorsement	
	Patients	Providers
I want [The patient wants] to get the recommended treatment	96.7	97.8
I believe [The patient believes] that the recommended treatment works (it helps to reduce my [his or her] symptoms)	90.0	97.8
The treatment worked while I [the patient] was at the NICoE so I [the patient] expect it will continue to work now	83.3	77.8
My [The patient's] spouse or partner encourages me [him or her] to get the recommended treatment (if applicable)	81.7	84.4
My providers [I] believe the recommended treatment works	60.0	86.7
My [The patient's] commander or supervisor supports me [him or her] getting the recommended treatment	55.0	88.9
The recommended treatment is easily accessible in my [the patient's] area	38.3	71.1
My doctor makes [I make] it mandatory for me [the patient] to receive the recommended treatment	31.7	22.2

NOTE: Percentages adjusted to exclude missing data.

riers to receiving NICoE recommended care were difficult scheduling an appointment (43 percent), concern that unit leadership might treat them differently (32 percent), concern that members of their unit might have less confidence in them (28 percent), and worry about being seen as weak (27 percent). Referring providers focused on a different set of barriers, noting the following: the patient not knowing where to get help (64 percent), patient difficulty getting time off work for the treatment (61 percent), and inadequate transportation (52 percent). Here again, providers were more likely to endorse barriers across the board compared to patients, but there were some particularly noticeable discrepancies as well. For example, while inadequate transportation was one of the barriers most commonly endorsed by providers, fewer than 2 percent of patients agreed that this was a barrier to care. Similarly, nearly half of providers thought that the patient's belief that the treatment would be ineffective was a barrier, while fewer than 2 percent of patients agreed. See Table 6.2 for all surveyed barriers and responses.

Consistent with survey responses to the barrier items, interviews with former NICoE patients also elicited evidence of limited availability of services at home stations. In some cases, patients noted that the recommended treatment simply isn't available:

> It was just, I did some different things, the water exercises, but where I'm at there's no swimming pool.

More often, former patients described a shortage of services and long wait times:

Table 6.2
Patient- and Home Station Provider–Identified Barriers to Receiving NICoE Recommended Care

Barriers to Care	Percent Endorsement	
	Patients	Providers
It is difficult [for the patient] to schedule an appointment	43.3	50.0
My [The patient's] unit leadership might treat me [him or her] differently	31.7	43.2
Members of my [the patient's] unit might have less confidence in me [him or her]	28.3	36.4
I [The patient] would be seen as weak	26.7	34.1
It would harm my [the patient's] career	25.0	27.3
There would be [The patient would have] difficulty getting time off work for treatment	21.7	61.4
My [The patient's] leaders would blame me [him or her] for the problem	21.7	25.0
TBI or psychological health care costs [the patient] too much money	15.0	6.8
I don't [The patient doesn't] trust TBI or psychological health professionals	13.3	50.0
I don't [The patient doesn't] know where to get help	13.3	63.6
It would be embarrassing [The patient would find it embarrassing]	10.0	31.8
I don't [The patient doesn't] have adequate transportation	1.7	52.3
[The patient believes] TBI or psychological health care doesn't work	1.7	47.7

NOTE: Percentages adjusted to exclude missing data.

My social worker says they are short on psychiatrists in [nearby city] so I didn't even get to see a psychiatrist until two months after I left NICoE.

Took them almost 9 months to get me back in to start seeing a counselor for my PTSD. Call to make an appointment, they'd call and say it was cancelled, send a re-schedule sheet. They'd apologize. Took me 9 months to get back in, but consistently seeing someone now in the past month.

Less commonly, patients described resistance from their providers in implementing NICoE recommendations:

Essentially [home station providers] thought it was a vacation, "That's what they do up there. Glad you had fun up there, but that's not how it works down here."

Patients had particular difficulty accessing recommended complementary and alternative medicine services noting that treatments such as acupuncture, massage therapy, and Botox are difficult to access in their area and, moreover, may not be covered by TRICARE.

A lot of the problem is once you get back home you can't get TRICARE to pay for the alternative treatments. It gets expensive when it's coming out of your pocket. They turn us loose with the whole treatment plan . . . but TRICARE won't pay for that when you get home.

Consistent with the experiences of patients, home station providers also noted limited access to specialty services. In some cases, this was due to limited availability of specialists. More often, providers mentioned insurance coverage problems, noting that TRICARE doesn't cover a particular treatment in their region (e.g., acupuncture). In fact, in response to a survey item assessing strategies to improve NICoE recommendations, a substantial majority of home station providers (89 percent) indicated that it was important that NICoE staff improve their "knowledge of the availability of specific types of services at the patient's home station."

During our discussions with NICoE staff, there was some evidence that they were, indeed, aware that resources are often limited at home stations and that TRICARE may not pay for NICoE recommendations to be implemented. During site visit interviews, NICoE staff made comments such as:

[We're] still sending them back to a place with very few resources, that's still the challenge.

Acupuncture is not a TRICARE covered benefit, that's when we start working with the case manager to identify local resources.

Some service members are lost to follow-up because they can't physically get to the appointment. Just being here and then going back is shock enough. If they're plugged in even with a good case manager, it is still difficult.

In general, there was some agreement across respondent types that home station access to NICoE-recommended services can be challenging for patients. Although patient self-advocacy skills may be an important facilitator, these strategies may go only so far in a system with a shortage of specialty providers. Given these challenges, the NICoE may wish to better coordinate care recommendations with the care patients could reasonably expect to access in their home stations or to provide alternate routes to obtaining recommended care. For example, patients and home station providers note that equipment procured during the NICoE stay (e.g., Continuous Positive Airway Pressure (CPAP) machines) facilitated continued use of this treatment on return to the home station.

Finally, it is worth noting that while stigma-related barriers to treatment were not offered during interviews, survey responses indicated that about one-quarter of patients had concerns about being seen as weak in the eyes of their leadership and colleagues. These stigma-related concerns may serve as a significant barrier to accessing care.

Patient Satisfaction with Home Station Care Following the NICoE

NICoE patients return home to a variety of treatment facilities. Given the diversity of home stations, it is perhaps not unexpected that satisfaction with home station care also varied. During interviews with former NICoE patients, some noted exceptional care on return to their home stations, and others were dissatisfied with home station services relative to the care they received at the NICoE. For example, one said:

> It's definitely made it easier back here. Right now I'm getting pretty good care. I can't say the same for people who have similar issues to me, and it's all because of NICoE.

Another patient had a different perspective:

> You make all of this progress at NICoE, and then you come back and stall. You go from extremely great care to nothing.

On the survey, former patients indicated their level of satisfaction with their home station care before they went to the NICoE, their satisfaction with the NICoE, and their satisfaction with home station care after they returned from the NICoE. Item response options ranged from 1 (not at all satisfied) to 5 (completely satisfied). As shown in Table 6.3, overall satisfaction with home station care after returning from the NICoE was moderate ($M = 2.6$)

Table 6.3
Patient Satisfaction with Care for TBI and Psychological Health

Satisfaction with	Pre-NICoE Home Station	NICoE	Post-NICoE Home Station
Overall care received	2.1 (1.18)$_a$	4.5 (0.67)$_b$	2.6 (1.18)$_c$
Care received to address main concern	1.8 (1.0)$_a$	4.5 (0.84)$_b$	2.7 (1.19)$_c$
Relationship with providers	2.5 (1.1)$_a$	4.7 (0.52)$_b$	3.0 (1.26)$_c$
Providers' knowledge of TBI/PH	2.2 (1.2)$_a$	4.8 (0.47)$_b$	2.9 (1.22)$_c$

NOTES: Across each row, values marked by different subscripts are statistically significantly different at the $p < 0.01$ level. Differences were tested with dependent-samples t-tests.
All items were measured on a 1 (not at all satisfied) to 5 (completely satisfied) scale.

but improved relative to satisfaction with pre-NICoE care (M=2.1, t [59] = 3.06, p < 0.01). Satisfaction with care at the NICoE was, on average, very high (M=4.5) and considerably higher than satisfaction with home station care either pre- or post-NICoE (ps < 0.01). In response to a question about whether the "trip to NICoE has positively influenced the treatment of my TBI and psychological health back home," 86 percent of former NICoE patients answered affirmatively. See Table 6.3 for complete results detailing patients' satisfaction with care for their primary concern, their relationship with their providers, and their providers' knowledge about TBI and PH.

Although home station providers often described positive aspects of their collaboration with the NICoE to improve patient care, many also noted that after a patient returns from the NICoE, the therapeutic relationship can be disrupted. For example:

> We've had problems with guys coming back very demanding and very entitled, yelling at our case managers. . . . We've had enough guys be flat out rude to case managers who are just trying to make the regular medical system work and it's just not good enough. That's been a consistent problem.

> NICoE seems to catastrophize that injury. The patients say: "Look—my TBI" [in a brain image]. Patients feel better when they can cling to something, but that doesn't generate progress and therapy. "Why bother, my brain will always be injured." That's what we hear coming from patients and that frustrates them. It goes against the message that we've been giving them. They are going to have that conflict, and who do you trust more? Splitting of the good versus bad. "[NICoE] is going to send me back to the bad" creates a therapeutic problem.

Overall, it appears that on average patients are slightly more satisfied with their home station care after their return from the NICoE, and, moreover, they believe their trip to the NICoE played a role in improving their care at home. However, comments from both patients and providers suggest a concern that there may be some splitting between NICoE staff and home station providers that may be leading to disruptions in the therapeutic alliance between former NICoE patients and their home station providers. It will be important that, even as NICoE takes a leadership role in the assessment of challenging cases, a collaborative relationship is maintained between providers working in both settings.

Conclusion

The NICoE's discharge planning process involves the collaboration of many specialists at the NICoE. Patients also provide input to the treatment plan. The NICoE staff reported they also consider the resources available at the patient's home station and try to write the discharge summary to be useful for both patient and provider audiences. Some home station providers may not be aware of these efforts, however, as several complained that the discharge summaries did not appear to acknowledge the treatment that had already been provided to the patient or the limited resources that would be available to the patient at the home station. Overall, patients, the NICoE, and some home station providers agreed that shortening the discharge summaries would be beneficial. Home station providers also indicated that they would like more direct communication from the NICoE about the patient and the treatment plan during and after the patient's stay there.

The NICoE often recommends a mix of traditional and complementary and alternative medicine approaches to treat patients' primary complaint. There was considerable variation in the extent to which home stations could implement the NICoE recommendations, with some stations easily offering all recommended treatments and others struggling to do so. Meeting recommendations for alternative and complementary approaches to care appeared particularly challenging, at least in part due to a shortage of providers and lack of coverage by TRICARE. However, even traditional specialty care appears difficult to access at some home stations with long wait times due to provider shortages. Patients were only moderately satisfied with their home station care, compared to high satisfaction with the NICoE services. However, it appears that average satisfaction with home station care may improve following stays at the NICoE, suggesting that some component of NICoE care may carry over to improve satisfaction with home station care (e.g., patient self-advocacy skills, explicit NICoE recommendations).

CHAPTER SEVEN

Discussion and Recommendations

The aims of this evaluation of the NICoE were to

- evaluate the process of referral of service members from the home station to the NICoE
- describe the NICoE assessment and treatment processes, including interactions with the home station during that time
- evaluate the patient's process of transitioning back to the home station and home station providers' implementation of the NICoE recommendations.

This chapter summarizes the key findings from the study and describes limitations that should be considered in interpreting our results. We conclude by offering suggestions for improving care for service members who are eligible to receive services at the NICoE.

Summary of Findings

The NICoE's History and Mission

NICoE staff described the center's mandate as one that seeks to "influence improvements in quality of care across the system," and the NICoE sees itself as a leader in developing TBI and psychological health evaluation and treatment approaches. However, there was some disagreement about whether the NICoE's mission and priorities had been clearly defined. Both NICoE staff and home station providers emphasized the importance of defining the roles and responsibilities of all providers at the outset.

Home station providers and patients perceived the NICoE role as mitigating some of the barriers service members face in seeking treatment for TBI or psychological health problems, including resource constraints, stigma, and provider turnover at home station facilities. There were differences in how home station providers viewed the role of the NICoE's diagnostic services. Providers at smaller, more rural sites viewed the NICoE's clinical role as extremely valuable. Providers from larger facilities were more likely to perceive the NICoE's role as duplicative and equivalent in quality. That said, most providers agreed that more communication and a better understanding of the NICoE's mission and services would help improve coordination among the facilities and providers involved with a patient's care.

Patients and their spouses were nearly unanimous in their praise of the NICoE's services, describing the extent to which the services and education received at the NICoE had helped them and, in some cases, contrasting the quality of these services with those offered at their home stations.

Referral of Service Members to the NICoE

The NICoE has advertised its eligibility criteria to include

- active-duty service members from any service branch (including the National Guard and reservists on orders)
- a mission-related mild or moderate TBI
- comorbid psychological health condition(s)
- failure to respond to TBI and mental health care offered at the service member's home station
- potential and desire to return to duty.

We found that the first four criteria are generally implemented by the NICoE, but the requirement of a potential and desire to return to duty is not (e.g., many patients are going through the medical evaluation board at the time of referral). Many providers we spoke with at site visits were uncertain about who should be referred to the NICoE. Provider survey respondents highlighted diagnostic complexity and nonresponse to previous treatment as the top reasons they refer to the NICoE. Many providers did not know how the NICoE decides which patients to accept and said they would appreciate feedback from the NICoE when it does not accept a patient. Some reported that special forces and higher-ranking service members seemed to be accepted more often than other service members. Overall, providers believed the referral process was relatively simple but thought it could be improved with an electronic referral option.

Former NICoE patients recalled that their pre-NICoE functioning was seriously impaired by their TBI and psychological health condition and that they were dissatisfied with the care they were receiving prior to the NICoE. They described disjointed and noncomprehensive care with long wait times and several weeks between appointments. Staff shortages were commonly blamed for these issues. Poor coordination between home station providers was also cited by patients as a reason for suboptimal care at their home stations prior to their time at the NICoE.

NICoE Assessment and Treatment Processes

In general, providers viewed the types of services offered at the home station to be similar to those offered at the NICoE, with the exception of alternative therapies and services for families. Patients' perceived gaps in care at home station facilities appear to be at least partially due to facility size and resources, including staffing levels. Some providers felt that patients tended to have a lower opinion of the services provided at their home station after receiving additional or different diagnostic information from the NICoE. In general, however, providers highlighted the individual attention that NICoE staff members are able to provide to patients and their families and rated patients' satisfaction with their stay at the NICoE as overwhelmingly positive.

Some providers also noted gaps in the way information about patient progress is shared while the patient is at the NICoE. Some felt that they could offer information about a patient's history and treatment but had not been included in initial meetings. Some providers also felt subordinate or dismissed by NICoE staff in discussing patients' care. This group confirmed that additional communication from the NICoE, including in-person meetings, would improve mutual understanding of the services provided at each facility.

The NICoE places a significant emphasis on education and the opportunity for family members to be informed and involved in a patient's care. Patients and their spouses had generally positive impressions of the NICoE's efforts, and we heard during our site visits that this type of engagement is not common at patients' home station facilities. We also heard from this group that communication could be improved prior to patients' admission to the NICoE, with more information about what to expect during the stay and a more clearly defined role for spouses who accompany patients.

Transitioning from the NICoE Back to the Home Station

Discharge planning at the NICoE involves an interdisciplinary team of NICoE staff, led by a primary care physician, and includes feedback and input from the patient and sometimes his or her spouse. The patient's home station providers are invited to participate in a call where the NICoE team presents the treatment plan and the home station provider can provide feedback and ask questions. Participating patients and home station providers appreciated having a voice in the discharge planning process.

The NICoE's assessment findings and recommended treatment plan are also synthesized in a comprehensive discharge summary. This summary, which is intended to integrate the findings and recommendations from all the specialists on the NICoE team and to be useful for both patients and providers, is challenging to construct and relatively long. While many providers and patients found the discharge summary very useful, we consistently heard that it would be easier to use if it were shorter. In addition, home station providers reported that the NICoE often seems to recommend the same treatment regimen that was provided prior to the NICoE. Some recommendations were difficult to implement given limited availability of resources at the home station.

Patients' and providers' views about patients' return to their home stations following care at the NICoE were mixed. Some experienced a smooth transition and a warm hand-off while others encountered problems accessing the recommended care. About half of participating former NICoE patients reported receiving post-NICoE care at an MTF; about a fifth reported receiving care at a VA and from civilian providers. Within these settings, service members were seeing a variety of "home station providers" for TBI-related care, most commonly primary care physicians, psychiatrists, and neurologists.

Both traditional and complementary and alternative medicine approaches to care were named as common NICoE recommendations. For the most part, the care NICoE providers recommended was reported to be relatively easy to implement. However, some home station providers noted that administrative hurdles posed a challenge, and they chose not to implement recommendations for care that the patient had already tried prior to his or her stay at the NICoE. NICoE staff noted that they would appreciate feedback from home station providers about implementation issues so that they could try to anticipate barriers to care and address them earlier in the process.

Patients and home station providers most commonly endorsed patient confidence in and desire for the recommended care as facilitators to obtaining the services NICoE recommended. Patients also highlighted communication and self-advocacy skills learned at the NICoE as important for obtaining services. The barrier to NICoE-recommended care most commonly reported by patients and by many providers was limited availability of recommended services at the home station and, relatedly, difficulty scheduling an appointment. This may be due to the limits of TRICARE coverage and also to a shortage of specialists in the patient's region.

Patients had very favorable views about the NICoE and were significantly less satisfied with the home station services they received before and after the NICoE. While post-NICoE care was reported retrospectively to be significantly better than pre-NICoE care overall, many service members, as noted previously, found it challenging to get the care they needed after the NICoE. Findings suggested that there may be some splitting between NICoE staff and home station providers that may disrupt the therapeutic alliance between former NICoE patients and their home station providers.

There was considerable variation in perceptions of the NICoE's recommendations. Patients were typically satisfied with the recommendations, but noted that their providers were not always supportive. Some providers had positive views about the NICoE's recommendations, while others said they are often duplicative of their original approach to care, or that when new recommendations are made by the NICoE, they reflect tertiary concerns that may not improve functioning.

Study Limitations

Study limitations should be considered when interpreting the results. First, the generalizability of our findings is limited. We did not survey or interview all former NICoE patients and their providers, and, thus, our sample may not be representative of the overall population of TBI patients and providers in the military. For instance, our findings could reflect only the opinions of those with strong (positive or negative) enough views about the NICoE to take time to participate. Although patient and provider survey response rates were only 20–30 percent, this is within the expected range for web surveys (Kaplowitz, Hadlock, and Levine, 2004), particularly considering that no incentives were provided. Similarly, we visited a limited number of home stations, and although we sought to maximize variability in experiences with the NICoE with our method of site selection, there may be opinions and experiences not represented in this evaluation. During site visits, spouses were invited to participate in discussions, but only four did so, which limits generalizability of our findings regarding spouse experiences.

Our data collection focused on providers and patients with some familiarity or experience with the NICoE. We cannot speculate on the extent to which our findings about home station TBI care generalize to service members with TBI who have not been referred to the NICoE, or to TBI providers with no knowledge of the NICoE or who are not working within the military health system. It is also possible that the overall positive views about the NICoE expressed by former NICoE patients were biased by patients' pretreatment expectations that the NICoE would provide higher-quality care than their home station. In particular, these positive expectancies could be due to a perception that more care is better care (Carman et al., 2010). We were not able to test this possibility in our evaluation, however.

This study was cross-sectional, retrospective, and used self-report methods. Any participant may have recall difficulties, but patients with TBI-related memory impairments may have particular difficulty accurately recalling past experiences. Future evaluations should implement prospective, longitudinal designs to more rigorously assess service members' transitions to and from the NICoE.

Although the NICoE is relatively well known among TBI providers in the MHS and has gained national attention (Martin, 2013), it had only been operational for four years at the time of this writing and has likely changed a great deal since its inception. There has been provider turnover at the NICoE and at home stations during that time, and the first cohort of NICoE patients likely had a different experience transitioning to and from the NICoE compared to more recent cohorts. Relationships and communication strategies between the NICoE and home stations may have changed over time, and our findings do not necessarily account for such adaptations, including those that have occurred since our data collection ended. Despite these limitations, we believe the integration of multiple data sources, both quantitative and qualitative, provides key insights about communication patterns between the NICoE and the home station providers and patient transitions between facilities.

Recommendations

In this section, we draw on key findings from the evaluation to provide recommendations to improve future care for service members with TBI. Following the organization of the report, we start with recommendations related to the NICoE's mission. We then present recommendations pertaining to the process of referring patients to the NICoE, the assessment and treatment services the NICoE provides, and the process by which patients transition back to their home stations.

The NICoE's Mission

Recommendation 1. Clearly define and communicate the clinical, research, and educational roles of the NICoE within the Military Health System (MHS). The NICoE's mission is to play a role in complex TBI treatment, research, and education, but for some NICoE staff and home station providers we spoke with, the role of the NICoE was not yet clear. Also, given increased attention and investment in TBI research and treatment within DoD, the VA, and civilian sectors (e.g., the National Institutes of Health), the assessment and treatment of TBI is likely to evolve and advance rapidly in the coming years. As such changes occur, input from home station providers at locations with and without satellites as well as from MHS policy and decisionmakers may be valuable in helping the NICoE determine its optimal role in caring for service members with TBI. We identified two specific recommendations in this area.

Recommendation 1a. Review and adapt the NICoE's strategic plan as the NICoE and the MHS evolve. To identify the optimal role for the NICoE and its satellite clinics within the MHS, both now and in the future, NICoE stakeholders should regularly review and consider potential adaptations to the NICoE's strategic plan. In doing so, stakeholders should consider the history of the NICoE, the changing context of the MHS (i.e., in light of the post-OEF/OIF drawdowns), and their vision for the NICoE over the next five or ten years. The strategic plan should also identify measurable goals for the NICoE, with a clear strategy for meeting those goals.

Recommendation 1b. Develop a consistent message about the role of the NICoE and disseminate this message widely. Once the optimal role for the NICoE is determined, the NICoE should clearly, broadly, and routinely disseminate its message about its role, as well as any changes to its policies and how it interacts with service members and home station providers. A strategic plan could be used as a guiding document for developing outreach and messaging materials. In addition, other DoD organizations that aim to improve care for service members with TBI and psychological health problems (e.g., DCoE, DVBIC) should collaborate with the NICoE to ensure that all entities are delivering a consistent and clear message about the NICoE's role to service members and their families, providers, and the public.

Recommendation 2. Foster a collaborative culture between the NICoE and home station providers. Some home station providers felt that their patients returned from the NICoE with negative opinions about the care they were previously receiving and mistrust for their home station providers, which interfered with their ability to work together and led some home station providers to resent the NICoE. NICoE and home station providers may have different treatment philosophies and models of care. However, they should work together to develop a clear and collaborative message about the roles of the NICoE and the home station.

Referral of Service Members to the NICoE

Recommendation 3. Inform home station providers about the NICoE's eligibility criteria. We identified three specific recommendations in this area.

Recommendation 3a. List and regularly update eligibility criteria on the NICoE referral form and website. Home station providers expressed confusion about the NICoE's inclusion and exclusion criteria. Eligibility criteria should be clearly stated on the NICoE referral form and on the NICoE website.

Recommendation 3b. Reconsider "potential and desire to return to active duty" as a NICoE eligibility criterion. This criterion appears to be in conflict with other eligibility criteria such as "failure to respond to TBI and mental health care offered at the service member's home station." Failure to respond to previous treatment could be due to the complexity and severity of a service member's condition, which may ultimately make him or her unlikely to return to full duty. Further, this criterion does not seem to be consistently implemented, as many NICoE patients reported being in the process of a Medical Evaluation Board review prior to and while at the NICoE. From a force strength perspective, it may be important to restrict access to the NICoE to only those service members who are most likely to return to active duty. If this is the priority, potentially conflicting eligibility criteria may need to be eliminated or revised for clarity.

Recommendation 3c. Adhere to eligibility criteria consistently and clearly communicate to home station providers the rationale for any exceptions or modifications. Eligibility criteria may evolve as the NICoE satellites open and as the needs of service members and the MHS change over time. Further, the NICoE may wish to actively recruit specific types of service members at times, such as those identified as underserved or those eligible for active research studies at the NICoE. Nonetheless, several patients and providers expressed frustration that certain types of service members (e.g., special forces, higher ranking) appeared to have an easier time getting into the NICoE than others. The NICoE should ensure that its intake and referral processes are as consistent, fair, and transparent as possible. When exceptions or revisions to eligibility criteria must be made, the rationale should be clearly communicated to home station providers. To facilitate transparency, the NICoE should consider publicly reporting data on the number of service members who were referred, accepted, and denied admission (and the reason) each year.

Recommendation 4. Focus patient recruitment on service members in greatest need. We identified two specific recommendations in this area.

Recommendation 4a. Actively seek referrals for service members at low-resource home stations. Many service members with TBI have little access to effective treatment due to their geographic location. Our findings suggest that the patients and providers who perceived the greatest benefit of the NICoE were those located at sites with few resources, geographically isolated from major hospitals and treatment centers. Outreach to providers and service members at Community Based Warrior Transition Units, civilian health centers serving large numbers of military personnel such as National Guard and reservists, and other nonmilitary treatment facility sites may bring the NICoE referrals and simultaneously help connect underserved service members with the TBI care they need. In addition to direct patient recruitment, NICoE outreach could include education about the NICoE and its services and consultation with home station providers. This could occur via in-person visits, telephone calls, emails, or mailings (e.g., brochures). If this recommendation is implemented, it will be important to carefully tailor the treatment plan for service members at these sites to ensure the availability of recommended care once they return to their home stations. In addition, unlike patients from high-resource stations, these patients may not have completed first-line CPG recommended treatments for TBI and comorbid mental health conditions (VA/DoD, 2009a; 2009b; 2010). Treatment plans should therefore focus on obtaining evidence-based care for these patients, as opposed to the alternative treatments more appropriate for those who have already tried and failed first-line care.

Recommendation 4b. In deciding which patients to accept at the NICoE, consider prioritizing service members who have very complex presentations or who have exhausted all home station treatment options. Some providers at high-resource sites (i.e., large military treatment facilities with specialized TBI clinics) said that the majority of services provided by the NICoE were available at the home station, and, therefore, they did not understand why some patients had gone to the NICoE. To conserve resources, the NICoE should consider a more conservative intake process, limiting referrals from high-resource home stations to only the most complex cases and those who have exhausted local treatment options. The NICoE could also offer consultation to home station providers treating patients with complex symptoms in need of certain expertise or a second opinion as a first step before accepting these patients into the NICoE.

NICoE Assessment and Treatment Services

Recommendation 5. Evaluate the effects of NICoE assessment and treatment services on patient outcomes. Many home station providers and some former NICoE patients questioned whether it was necessary for the NICoE's services to be so comprehensive, devoting resources to identifying and treating problems without obvious connections to the TBI. Furthermore, some study participants (both patients and providers) suggested that the act of traveling to a different place, escaping day-to-day hassles to focus on oneself, explained the improvement in patient symptoms and wondered whether treatment gains could be sustained over time. Future studies using experimental designs or matched comparison groups may help determine the extent to which NICoE services result in improved patient outcomes (e.g., TBI symptom reduction, occupational functioning) compared with treatment as usual (e.g., at a home station TBI clinic). To best measure this effect, we recommend randomized controlled trials, in which patients are randomly assigned to each treatment condition. However, if such a study is impractical, a comparative effectiveness approach to examine the added benefit of the NICoE compared with usual care would be a valuable alternative.

Recommendation 5a. Conduct a cost analysis of the NICoE. As the NICoE represents a considerable investment of resources, an analysis should be conducted to determine the costs associated with providing services to service member populations at the NICoE compared with home stations and to identify which services could be provided at home stations for the same or lower cost. Results from an outcome evaluation could be incorporated into a cost analysis as well to determine the cost-effectiveness of the NICoE compared to usual care. We note that any cost analysis should take into account the unique nature of the NICoE as a public-private partnership.

Transitioning from the NICoE Back to the Home Station

Recommendation 6. Increase and formalize communication and coordination between the NICoE and home station providers. We identified two specific recommendations in this area.

Recommendation 6a. Bolster communication and coordination early on in the treatment process (ideally at intake) and sustain this level throughout the patient's stay at the NICoE. The amount of communication and coordination between home station and NICoE staff prior to discharge appeared to be related to the level of home station provider satisfaction with the discharge process overall. Home station providers who had been in contact with NICoE staff prior to and during the discharge process reported finding those interactions valuable in helping them understand the progress made at the NICoE and in planning for follow-up care at the home station. Currently, the NICoE communicates with the referring home station provider primarily at intake and discharge and not as much throughout the patient's stay at the NICoE. To improve communication, the NICoE may wish to coordinate the time of these calls with home station providers' schedules to increase the likelihood that the home station provider can attend.

Recommendation 6b. Enhance communication between the NICoE and home station specialty providers. Given that the NICoE is unusual in its integrated interdisciplinary approach to care, we suggest connecting specialists with one another. Improved information sharing may also allow the NICoE to ensure that all treating home station providers—not just the referring provider—are invited to the discharge conference call and directly sent the discharge summary.

Recommendation 7. Streamline discharge summaries and provide recommendations in the context of the treatment already delivered by the home station. We identified two specific recommendations in this area.

Recommendation 7a. List treatment recommendations near the beginning of the report. Several patients and providers noted the NICoE discharge summary is somewhat cumbersome due to its length. They mentioned that the summary would be more helpful if there were a "bottom line up front." For instance, recommendations could be listed on the first page rather than the last page.

Recommendation 7b. Ensure that discharge summaries clearly acknowledge services previously delivered and provide a rationale. Home station providers noted that NICoE treatment recommendations sometimes suggested treatment modes that have already been completed or were ineffective. These providers were uncertain as to whether this was because NICoE providers were unaware of the services previously delivered or because they believed more of that treatment—or a different version of it—would be helpful. In such cases, NICoE providers should explicitly acknowledge previous treatment when they are aware of it and explain the reasoning for suggesting more of the same intervention.

Recommendation 8. Ensure that service members can access recommended care at or near their home station and are aware of its cost. The CAM approaches offered by the NICoE were commonly recommended but often difficult to access at service members' home stations. Some former NICoE patients said they were frustrated and surprised to learn that

CAM and other nontraditional treatments (e.g., Botox for headaches) that helped them at the NICoE were not covered by TRICARE. Participants appreciated the NICoE's existing efforts to avert such barriers. For instance, the NICoE sends some patients with sleep apnea home with a CPAP machine so that they do not have to devote time to obtaining one on their own. Before completing the discharge summary, the NICoE should work with the patient and with home station providers to determine (1) whether specific services are available at or near the home station and (2) whether they are covered by the service member's insurance. When a treatment is not covered or easily accessible (e.g., no providers within reasonable driving distance or very long wait lists), the team should prepare a backup plan. For instance, the NICoE could specifically recommend that CAM approaches such as yoga, meditation, and guided relaxation be accessed online and provide the relevant web links in the discharge summary.

Recommendation 9. Enhance patient tracking and follow-up after discharge. According to participating NICoE staff members, the NICoE aims to follow all of its patients indefinitely after they are discharged to determine whether treatment gains are sustained and whether patients are accessing needed care, as well as to identify gaps in services or barriers to care that must be addressed. However, as the number of NICoE alumni grows over time, this will become unmanageable for the (at the time of our study) one individual assigned to this task. While it may seem that using AHLTA for this purpose would make sense, it is currently infeasible; the system, used by the NICoE to track patients, is stored only at the NICoE and is inaccessible to other providers who may have valuable information to contribute or who may be able to use the information the NICoE collects about its patients to improve home station care. To successfully follow patients after discharge and identify barriers to care and gaps in services, more resources must be invested in this effort, both in terms of manpower and in devising a better method for patient follow-up. There has been some discussion of using a TBI registry administered by DVBIC, and integrating NICoE patient follow-up data into this or another system is one option to explore (Langlois and Rutland-Brown, 2005).

Conclusion

This report offered a general overview of the NICoE referral and discharge processes from the perspectives of NICoE staff, home station providers, and former NICoE patients and their spouses. We also reviewed the services provided at the NICoE. Based on input from web surveys and during site visit interviews, our recommendations focus on improving communication and clarifying the NICoE's role in relation to home station treatment facilities. The recommendations address some of the common challenges cited by survey and interview participants and include revisions to the eligibility criteria and the extent to which they are enforced, suggestions for improving patient selection to ensure that resources are allocated efficiently, and options to strengthen communication, coordination, and follow-up treatment during and after a patient's stay at the NICoE.

NICoE Site Visit Discussion Guide

Verbal Consent for Discussions

The RAND Corporation, a nonprofit research organization, is conducting a study funded by the Defense Centers of Excellence (DCoE) for Psychological Health and Traumatic Brain Injury (TBI) to better understand programs identified as innovative or promising. NICoE was selected as one of these. We are interested in talking with you to learn more about the roles and responsibilities of NICoE providers/staff relative to the providers/staff at a service member's home base. We are also interested in learning more about recommendations and communication patterns between a service member's NICoE providers/staff and home station providers/staff. Your participation in this study is entirely voluntary and confidential. RAND will use the information you provide for research purposes only, and will not disclose your identity or information that identifies you to anyone outside the project team. We will be taking notes and audio recording our conversation today. During the course of the study, we will safeguard this information, and after the study is complete, we will destroy all recordings. You are under no obligation to discuss anything that you do not feel comfortable discussing with me and should feel free to decline to answer any question that you do not wish to answer. We estimate that our discussion will take about one hour.

For more information about this study, please contact either Gery Ryan or Carrie Farmer by phone at (310) 393-0411. If you have any questions about your rights as a research participant, you may contact Carolyn Tschopik, Administrator, RAND Human Subjects Protection Committee by phone at (310) 393-0411 or by email: tschopik@rand.org.

Do you have any questions before we begin?

Do you agree to participate in this interview?

No » Okay, thank you for your time.

Yes » Thank you very much. We really appreciate your support.

Discussion Prompts

As I mentioned before, our task is to document patterns of coordination and communication between patients' home station treatment providers/staff and their NICoE providers/staff. We'd like to cover three points in the timeline. First, we're hoping to learn more about the referral process. Second, we're interested in learning more about your interactions with home station providers/staff while a patient is being treated at NICoE. Finally, we'd like to talk with you about coordinating a patient's transition back to the care of home station providers and the long-term treatment plans that NICoE develops for patients.

Providers

Referral/Intake process

- I'd like to start at the beginning of the referral process (i.e., before a patient has been accepted for treatment at NICoE). Please tell me about the information that is typically provided to NICoE from home station providers?
    - What is the intake process like? (Describe interactions w/ providers, types of providers, info typically provided w/ referral.)
    - How is this information typically exchanged?
    - What have patients' experiences been like pre-NICoE?
    - What are the most common reasons patients are referred to NICoE?

- How many patients are referred to NICoE?
    - How does NICoE determine who will be accepted into the program and when?
    - What are the eligibility criteria?

        Variables of interest:
        ○ Screening procedures (how is patient eligibility determined?)
        ○ Assessment procedures, types (e.g., how many Posttraumatic Stress Disorder Checklist (PCLs) given per month?)
        ○ Treatment procedures, types (e.g., how many patients get family therapy?)
        ○ Where are the referrals from?
        ○ To where does NICoE typically refer patients after completion?
        ○ Patient characteristics: demographics, military occupational specialty (MOS), service, deployment history, diagnoses, pre-NICoE treatment history, NICoE treatment recommendations, post-NICoE treatment received?

- What role do the NICoE satellite locations play in the referral process?
- What are the barriers and facilitators of a smooth referral process?
- How many patients can receive treatment at the NICoE at one time?
    - How long is the waitlist?
- What are most common diagnoses/problems?
- What is working well?
- What could be improved?

I'd like to transition to some questions about your interactions with home station providers/staff while a patient is being treated by NICoE and after he or she returns home. Before I do, is there anything more you'd like to share about the referral process before I move on?

At NICoE

- Once a patient arrives at NICoE, what evaluation and treatment services are provided and how is the protocol determined? *(NOTE: DROP QUESTION AFTER SATURATION IS REACHED)*
- How is the recommended treatment plan determined? Who is involved in that process?
  - [IF NOT OFFERED] To what extent do the patient's home station providers contribute to the treatment plan?
  - [IF NOT OFFERED] What role do patients and their families play in this process?
    - For example, how often is it necessary to rely upon caregiver/spouse reports due to memory or other impairment from service members' brain injuries?
- How is progress tracked/monitored? (Do they have an electronic system/database to monitor symptoms? How often do they assess symptoms and with what measures?)
- What happens when NICoE's diagnostic findings are inconsistent with what was given by home station providers?
- After a treatment plan has been created, how is it communicated to home station providers?
  - How is it communicated to patients and their families?
- What are the barriers and facilitators of effective coordination between NICoE and home station providers regarding the patient's treatment plan?
  - Between NICoE and satellite locations?
- How common is it for the referring provider/treatment team to be the same provider/team to which the patient returns after NICoE?
- What is your impression of whether or not treatment plan recommendations are implemented by home station providers?
- What kinds of feedback is NICoE currently getting from base providers? From patients? From patient's families?

Discharge planning

- What considerations are made in discharge planning? (e.g., services available at the patient's installation, chain of command support for patient getting treatment)
- How is the report constructed?
- How is the patient and family informed of results, recommendations, etc.?
- Are NICoE follow-up calls or appointments scheduled?
  - Who makes follow-up appointments at the home station?

Post-NICoE follow-up

- How are patients tracked after leaving NICoE?
- What helps or hinders NICoE in tracking patients?
- What seems to help or hinder patients in getting care they need once back at home station?
- Do patients ever return to NICoE?

Overall mission/purpose of NICoE

- How prevalent is telemedicine?

Administrators

Referral/Intake process

- I'd like to start at the beginning of the referral process (i.e., before a patient has been accepted for treatment at NICoE). Please tell me about the information that is typically provided to NICoE from home station providers.
  - What is the intake process like? (Describe interactions w/ providers, types of providers, info typically provided w/ referral.)
  - How is this information typically exchanged?
  - What have patients' experiences been like pre-NICoE?
  - What are the most common reasons patients are referred to NICoE?

- How many patients are referred to NICoE?
  - How does NICoE determine who will be accepted into the program and when?
  - What are the eligibility criteria?

    Variables of interest:
    ○ Screening procedures (how is patient eligibility determined?)
    ○ Assessment procedures, types (e.g., how many Posttraumatic Stress Disorder Checklist (PCLs) given per month?)
    ○ Treatment procedures, types (e.g., how many patients get family therapy?)
    ○ Where are the referrals from?
    ○ To where does NICoE typically refer patients after completion?
    ○ Patient characteristics: demographics, military occupational specialty (MOS), service, deployment history, diagnoses, pre-NICoE treatment history, NICoE treatment recommendations, post-NICoE treatment received?

- What role do the NICoE satellite locations play in the referral process?
- What are the barriers and facilitators of a smooth referral process?
- How many patients can receive treatment at the NICoE at one time?
  - How long is the waitlist?

- What are most common diagnoses/problems?
- What is working well?
- What could be improved?

I'd like to transition to some questions about your interactions with home station providers/staff while a patient is being treated by NICoE and after he or she returns home. Before I do, is there anything more you'd like to share about the referral process before I move on?

At NICoE

- Once a patient arrives at NICoE, what evaluation and treatment services are provided and how is the protocol determined? *(NOTE: DROP QUESTION AFTER SATURATION IS REACHED)*
- How is the recommended treatment plan determined? Who is involved in that process?
  - [IF NOT OFFERED] To what extent do the patient's home station providers contribute to the treatment plan?
  - [IF NOT OFFERED] What role do patients and their families play in this process?

    ○ For example, how often is it necessary to rely upon caregiver/spouse reports due to memory or other impairment from service members' brain injuries?

- How is progress tracked/monitored? (Do they have an electronic system/database to monitor symptoms? How often do they assess symptoms and with what measures?)
- What happens when NICoE's diagnostic findings are inconsistent with what was given by home station providers?
- After a treatment plan has been created, how is it communicated to home station providers?
  - How is it communicated to patients and their families?
- What are the barriers and facilitators of effective coordination between NICoE and home station providers regarding the patient's treatment plan?
  - Between NICoE and satellite locations?
- How common is it for the referring provider/treatment team to be the same provider/team to which the patient returns after NICoE?
- What is your impression of whether or not treatment plan recommendations are implemented by home station providers?
- What kinds of feedback is NICoE currently getting from base providers? From patients? From patient's families?

Discharge planning

- What considerations are made in discharge planning? (e.g., services available at the patient's installation, chain of command support for patient getting treatment)
- How is the report constructed?
- How is the patient and family informed of results, recommendations, etc.?
- Are NICoE follow-up calls or appointments scheduled?
  - Who makes follow-up appointments at the home station?

Post-NICoE follow-up

- How are patients tracked after leaving NICoE?
- What helps or hinders NICoE in tracking patients?
- What seems to help or hinder patients in getting care they need once back at home station?

- Do patients ever return to NICoE?

Overall mission/purpose of NICoE

- What are the main objectives of NICoE?
  - How is NICoE monitored in its progress toward these objectives?
- How many staff are at the NICoE? (break down into clinical, administrative, research?)
- How (if at all) does military/DoD leadership (e.g., Regional Medical Commands, DVBIC, MTF commands, etc.) help or hinder NICoE in achieving its objectives?
- What is the current plan for satellites?
  - What has helped or hindered NICoE in getting satellites up and running?
- How prevalent is telemedicine?

Home Station Installation Patient Discussion Guide

I. Welcome participants.

II. Describe study, structure of a focus group, confidentiality and confidentiality safeguards. Emphasize need for all group members to protect the confidentiality of other group members by not sharing information they hear today.

III. Read verbal informed consent forms and respond to questions.

IV. **[Skip this step if conducting individual interview only]** Hand out questionnaire with open-ended questions about the treatment experiences prior to NICoE, at NICoE, and after returning to their home base following care at NICoE, including demographic items.

V. Use discussion guide to structure conversation allowing participants to take the lead when appropriate (i.e., broach new topics, discuss subareas of a given prompt).

Discussion Prompts

Thank you all for taking time out of your busy schedules to meet with us today. We'd like to cover three main topics today. First, we'd like to hear about how you first learned about NICoE and the referral process. Second, we'd like to hear about your care while you were at NICoE. And finally, we're hoping to get a better understanding of how your care did (or did not) change when you returned to your home station.

We'd like to keep the focus of the conversation on your experiences with medical and mental health care and barriers to care. We'll avoid talking about your medical or mental health diagnoses. This will help protect your confidentiality.

1. Before you went to NICoE, how were you functioning at that time? What challenges were you facing?

2. **[Verbally ask this question for individual interviews only]** Before you came to NICoE, what kinds of services or treatments were you receiving for TBI and other conditions (e.g., therapies, specialist doctors)? How long had you been in treatment?

3. What was your reaction when your doctor or therapist first told you about NICoE?

4. Can you talk a little about the process of coming to the decision to travel to D.C. to receive NICoE services?

5.   What was your time like at NICoE? What worked well for you and what didn't work well?

6.   How involved (if at all) were you in the treatment plan for your care after you left NICoE? What did you expect would happen when you got home in terms of your care?

7.   When you returned to your home base after being at NICoE, how did your care change (if at all) from what you were receiving before you went to NICoE? To what extent did your experiences at NICoE change how you thought about your care at home?

8.   To what degree do you feel your NICoE providers communicated what they learned about you and your condition to your home base providers? How could you tell?

9.   **[Verbally ask this question for individual interviews only]** What suggestions do you have to improve the services you received when you returned to your home base?

10. How are you doing now in terms of the care you are receiving? What challenges (if any) are you facing in getting the care that you think you need?

11. Transitioning from one set of doctors and therapists to a new facility and then back home again can be challenging; what advice would you give to a service member who is considering traveling to NICoE?

12. Do you think you are worse off, the same, or better off than you would have been if you had not traveled to NICoE?

13. **[Verbally ask this question for individual interviews only]** What were the most positive things that happened to you as a result of your involvement with NICoE?

14. **[Verbally ask this question for individual interviews only]** What suggestions do you have to improve NICoE services?

Home Station Installation Spouse/Caregiver Discussion Guide

I.   Welcome participants.

II. Describe study, structure of a focus group, confidentiality and confidentiality safeguards. Emphasize need for all group members to protect the confidentiality of other group members by not sharing information they hear today.

III. Read verbal informed consent forms and respond to questions.

IV. **[Skip this step if conducting individual interview only]** Hand out questionnaire with open-ended questions about the treatment experiences prior to NICoE, at NICoE, and after returning to their home base following care at NICoE, including demographic items.

V.   Use discussion guide to structure conversation allowing participants to take the lead when appropriate (i.e., broach new topics, discuss subareas of a given prompt).

Discussion Prompts

Thank you all for taking time out of your busy schedules to meet with us today. We'd like to cover three main topics today. First, we'd like to hear about how you first learned about NICoE and the referral process. Second, we'd like to hear about the care your spouse or family member received while he or she was at NICoE. And finally, we're hoping to get a better understanding of how his or her care did (or did not) change when they returned to your home station.

We'd like to keep the focus of the conversation on your experiences with medical and mental health care and barriers to care. We'll avoid talking about your spouse or family member's medical or mental health diagnoses. This will help protect his or her confidentiality.

1.   Before your service member went to NICoE, how were they functioning at that time? What challenges were they facing?

2.   Before your service member traveled to NICoE, what kinds of services or treatments was your service member receiving at your home station (e.g., therapies, specialist doctors)? How long had he or she been in treatment?

3.   **[Verbally ask this question for individual interviews only]** How did you come to learn about NICoE? What was your reaction?

4. Can you talk a little about the process of coming to the decision to travel to D.C. so your service member could receive NICoE services?

5. What was your time like at NICoE? What worked well for your spouse or family member and what didn't work well?

6. How involved (if at all) were you in the treatment plan for your service member's care after they left NICoE? What did you expect would happen when you got home in terms of their care?

7. When you returned to your home base after being at NICoE, how did your spouse or family member's care change (if at all) from what he or she was receiving before they went to NICoE? To what extent did your experiences at NICoE change how you thought about their care at home?

8. To what degree do you feel that the NICoE providers communicated what they learned about your service member and his or her condition to the home base providers? How could you tell?

9. **[Verbally ask this question for individual interviews only]** What suggestions do you have to improve the services your family member received at your home base?

10. How is your service member doing now in terms of the care they are receiving? What challenges (if any) are you facing in getting the care that you think he or she needs?

11. Transitioning from one set of doctors and therapists to a new facility and then back home again can be challenging, what advice would you give to a family member who is considering traveling to NICoE to support their service member?

12. Do you think your service member is worse off, the same, or better off than they would have been if they had not traveled to NICoE?

13. **[Verbally ask this question for individual interviews only]** What were the most positive things that you observed in your service member after he or she was a patient at NICoE?

14. **[Verbally ask this question for individual interviews only]** What suggestions do you have to improve NICoE services?

Home Station Installation Provider Discussion Guide

NICoE Evaluation Discussion Guide for MTF Providers

Opening script and consent procedure	Good morning/afternoon. My name is ___, and I am a researcher at the RAND Corporation, which is a nonprofit, nonpartisan policy research organization. I am going to lead the interview. My colleague ___ will take notes so that we are sure we accurately hear what you have to say but will not be participating in the discussion. We really appreciate your taking the time to share your input with us. RAND is conducting a research study to assess the National Intrepid Center of Excellence (NICoE) in Bethesda, Md. The study is funded by the DoD Defense Center of Excellence for Psychological Health and Traumatic Brain Injury (DCoE) and will examine communication patterns between service members' home station treatment teams and their NICoE treatment teams. We are interested in talking with you to learn more about how you decide to refer a patient to NICoE and your experiences with NICoE treatment recommendations for service members who return to your care. Your participation in this study is entirely voluntary and confidential. RAND will use the information you provide for research purposes only, and will not disclose your identity or information that identifies you to anyone outside the project team. We will be taking notes of our conversation today. During the course of the study, we will safeguard this information, and after the study is complete, we will destroy all notes. You are under no obligation to discuss anything that you do not feel comfortable discussing with me and should feel free to decline to answer any question that you do not wish to answer. We estimate that our discussion will take about one hour. Are you willing to participate in this interview? If yes, continue with script If no: "Okay, thank you for your time."
Overview	As I mentioned before, our task is to document patterns of coordination and communication between Bethesda-NICoE providers and the treatment team at the service member's home station. We'd like to cover three points in the timeline. First, we're hoping to learn more about the process of referring a patient to NICoE and how you come to the decision to do so. Second, we're interested in learning more about your interactions with NICoE staff while one of your patients is being treated there. Finally, we'd like to talk with you about your interactions with NICoE after a patient returns to your care and your experiences with the treatment plans that NICoE develops for patients. If you've never referred a patient to NICoE, we'd still like to hear about your impressions of the organization. Do you have any questions before we begin? [Answer questions.]
Introduction	To start, I'd like to hear about the kinds of patients you treat. Can you tell me a little about your typical caseload of patients? To what extent do you see or treat patients with a TBI and psychological health conditions such as PTSD?

Knowledge of NICoE

Next, I'd like to find out what you know about the National Intrepid Center of Excellence (NICoE) in Bethesda. Have you ever heard of NICoE?
How did you come to learn about NICoE and its mission?
Have you ever referred patients to NICoE?
[If never referred] Have you ever been assigned patients while they were at NICoE or after they were discharged from NICoE?
- If YES, go to Treatment section
- If NO, go to No Experience section

Referral

How do you determine which patients to refer to NICoE?
- [INTERVIEWER'S NOTE: You're trying to get them to tell you their perception of the eligibility criteria without leading.]
Are patients who are involved in a Physical Evaluation Board (PEB) referred? Why or why not?
At what point in a patient's care do you start to consider referring them to NICoE?
- [INTERVIEWER'S NOTE: Do they volunteer that treatment non-responsiveness is important?]
How do your patients typically respond when you bring up the possibility of receiving treatment at NICoE?
Describe the process of making a referral to NICoE.
- PROBE: What is the interviewee's role in the referral process?
How often are the patients who you refer to NICoE accepted?
- PROBE: IF LESS THAN 100%, Why did NICoE not accept some of your patients?
What kinds of interactions have you had with NICoE during the process of referring your patients?
What are the barriers to a successful referral? What are the facilitators to a successful referral?
I'd like to transition to some questions about your interactions with NICoE while your patient is being treated there and after your patient returns to your care. Before I do, is there anything more that you'd like to share about the referral process before we move on?

Treatment during/post NICoE

OK, now I'd like to ask about your experience treating patients while they are at NICoE and when they return from NICoE.
Typically, how involved are you in the development of the NICoE treatment plan?
When a patient returns to your care after being treated at NICoE, how does that transition occur? How much and what type of communication is there between NICoE and your facility?
Do your patients talk to you about their time at NICoE?
- [IF YES] What has been their impression of their time at the NICoE?
What is your impression of the treatment recommendations developed at NICoE?
To what extent (if at all) do you typically change your treatment plan in response to NICoE's recommendations?
How do you prioritize which NICoE treatment recommendations to implement?
What are the barriers to implementing their recommendations? What are the facilitators to implementing their recommendations?
In your experience, do patients who are treated at NICoE tend to get better as a result of going to NICoE? Why or why not?
Do your patients who are treated at the NICoE remain active duty?
- PROBE: What proportion stay active duty versus med board out of the service?

If no NICoE experience

What is your understanding of the services offered by the NICoE?
To what extent do these services seem relevant for the patients who you see?
In what circumstances would you consider referring a patient to the NICoE?
What things make you reluctant to send a patient to the NICoE?
What advice do you have for the NICoE as they work to improve their services?

Wrap-up

We're almost done, but before we finish, we'd like to hear your ideas for what NICoE could do to improve their services.
[For providers with NICoE experience] What advice do you have for NICoE to improve their referral process, evaluation and treatment of patients, or recommendations for care?
Is there anything else that you would like to say about this topic before we wrap up?

End

That's all the questions about NICoE that we have for you. Thank you so much for participating in this discussion; your feedback has been extremely valuable.
Here is my card with my contact information if you'd like more information or think of anything else you'd like to share. [Hand card]
Thanks again for your time.

Survey Measures

Provider Survey

Survey Item	Response Options	Source/Reference
Have you ever heard of the National Intrepid Center of Excellence (NICoE)?	0 No 1 Yes	N/A
Do you see patients with Traumatic Brain Injury (TBI) or psychological health conditions?	0 No 1 Yes	N/A
What is the highest level of education you have achieved?	1 High school diploma or GED 2 Some college 3 Associate's degree 4 Bachelor's degree 5 Master's degree 6 Doctoral degree (e.g., M.D., Ph.D., Psy.D., Ed.D.) 7 Other (please describe): _____	N/A
Are you currently…(select all that apply)	a. Active-duty military b. Reserve c. National Guard d. Civilian practitioner e. DoD employee f. Retired military g. Other (please specify):_____	N/A
[IF Military]: Of which service are/were you a member?	a. Air Force b. Army c. Coast Guard d. Marine Corps e. Navy	N/A
[IF Military]: What is/was your rank/rate/pay grade?	E1–E9 WO1/WO–CW5/CWO5 O1–O10	N/A

Survey Item	Response Options	Source/Reference
What is your primary discipline?	a. Clinical Psychology b. Neurology c. Neuropsychology d. Occupational Therapy e. Physical Therapy f. Primary Care Physician (Family Practice/ General Internal Medicine) g. Psychiatry h. Social Work i. Speech Therapy j. Other (please specify): _____	N/A
For how many years have you been evaluating and/ or treating patients with TBI and co-occurring psychological health disorders?	0–100, N/A	N/A
Thinking of your typical caseload, what percentage of your patients have a TBI or a psychological health disorder?	0–100%, N/A	N/A
How did you find out about the NICoE?	a. A patient b. My supervisor c. A colleague d. A training/workshop e. A research article, publication, or conference presentation f. National or local media (e.g., television, newspaper, radio) g. Other: _____	N/A
In what capacity have you had contact with the NICoE? *(check all that apply)*	a. I have referred patients to the NICoE b. I have seen patients who had previously been to the NICoE c. Neither of these	N/A
I have referred _____ patients to the NICoE.	[Fill in blank]	N/A
Of the patients I referred to the NICoE, _____ were accepted into the program.	[Fill in blank]	N/A
Of the patients I referred to the NICoE, _____ turned down an opportunity to go to the program.	[Fill in blank]	N/A
I have evaluated or treated _____ patients who had been discharged from the NICoE.	[Fill in blank]	N/A
[IF referred or treated more than one patient who attended the NICoE]: In general, how satisfied are you with the diagnostic evaluations your patient(s) received from the NICoE?	a. Not at all satisfied b. Slightly satisfied c. Moderately satisfied d. Very satisfied e. Completely satisfied	N/A

Survey Item	Response Options	Source/Reference
I would refer a patient to the NICoE if... (*check all that apply*)	a. The patient has a documented diagnosis of a mild or moderate TBI b. The patient has a documented psychological health disorder (e.g., depression, PTSD) c. The patient has insufficient access to necessary resources, treatment, or assessment d. The patient has the potential and desire to return to duty e. The patient's TBI or psychological health problems are very complex or severe f. The patient's symptoms are not improving with the current treatment g. Other (please explain): _____	N/A
I would *not* refer a patient to the NICoE if.... (*check all that apply*)	a. The patient does not have a history of TBI and co-occurring psychological diagnosis b. The patient's condition did not seem severe enough c. The patient was responding well to the treatment I was providing d. The patient told me s/he did not have the desire to return to duty e. The patient appeared to lack potential to return to duty f. The patient had access to the necessary assessment and treatment elsewhere g. The patient has an active substance abuse problem h. The patient recently completed inpatient or substance abuse treatment i. The patient isn't able to independently perform activities of daily living j. The patient does not have the capacity to engage safely in an intensive outpatient setting k. I believed the patient would receive better care at his or her home installation l. Other (please explain): _____	N/A
[IF has referred at least one patient to the NICoE]: In deciding whether to refer patients to the NICoE, do you consult with any of the following providers? (*check all the apply*)	a. Case manager b. Neurologist c. Nursing staff member d. Occupational therapist e. Physical therapist f. Primary care doctor g. Psychiatrist h. Psychologist i. Speech/language therapist j. Other (please explain): _____ k. I do not consult with other providers when considering a referral to the NICoE	N/A
[IF has referred at least one patient to the NICoE]: How likely are you to refer another patient to the NICoE?	a. Not at all b. Somewhat c. Moderately d. Very e. Extremely	N/A

Survey Item	Response Options	Source/Reference
[IF has seen at least one patient after NICoE discharge]: Based on your experiences with the NICoE, please indicate your level of satisfaction with the following:		N/A
Frequency of NICoE's communication with you about the patient	1 Not at all satisfied 2 Slightly satisfied 3 Moderately satisfied 4 Very satisfied 5 Completely satisfied	
Quality of NICoE's communication with you about the patient	1 Not at all satisfied 2 Slightly satisfied 3 Moderately satisfied 4 Very satisfied 5 Completely satisfied	
NICoE's referral process	1 Not at all satisfied 2 Slightly satisfied 3 Moderately satisfied 4 Very satisfied 5 Completely satisfied	
NICoE's recommendations	1 Not at all satisfied 2 Slightly satisfied 3 Moderately satisfied 4 Very satisfied 5 Completely satisfied	
[IF has seen at least one patient after NICoE discharge]: Have you ever read a NICoE discharge summary?	0. No 1. Yes	N/A
[IF has read a NICoE discharge summary]: How would you prefer to access the discharge summary? (*check all that apply*)	a. Patient records (e.g., AHLTA) b. NICoE sends it to me directly c. I have a phone conversation with the NICoE about the summary d. The patient shares it with me e. Other (please explain): _____	N/A
[IF has read a NICoE discharge summary]: To what extent does the NICoE discharge summary:		N/A
Improve your understanding of the patient's TBI and psychological health condition(s)?	1 Not at all 2 Somewhat 3 Moderately 4 Very much 5 Extremely	
Influence the treatment you provide to the patient?	1 Not at all 2 Somewhat 3 Moderately 4 Very much 5 Extremely	

Survey Item	Response Options	Source/Reference
Please rate the extent to which you agree or disagree that the following help your patients get the treatment or services NICoE recommends? .	(See below for response options to statements below.)	Britt, T. W., T. M. Greene-Shortridge, S. Brink, Q. B. Nguyen, J. Rath, A. L. Cox, C. W. Hoge, and C. A. Castro, Perceived Stigma and Barriers to Care for Psychological Treatment: Implications for Reactions to Stressors in Different Contexts, *Journal of Social and Clinical Psychology*, Vol. 27, 2008, pp. 317–335. Schell, Terry L., and Grant N. Marshall, "Survey of Individuals Previously Deployed for OEF/OIF," in Tanielian, Terri L., Lisa H. Jaycox, Terry L. Schell, Grant N. Marshall, M. Audrey Burnam, Christine Eibner, Benjamin R. Karney, Lisa S. Meredith, Jeanne S. Ringel, and Mary E. Vaiana, eds., *Invisible Wounds of War: Summary and Recommendations for Addressing Psychological and Cognitive Injuries*, Santa Monica, CA: RAND Corporation, MG-720/1-CCF, 2008. As of July 25, 2014: http://www.rand.org/pubs/monographs/MG720z1.html
a. The treatment is easily accessible in the patient's area.	1 Strongly Disagree 2 Disagree 3 Neither Disagree nor Agree 4 Agree 5 Strongly Agree	
b. The patient's commander or supervisor supports him or her getting the treatment.	1 Strongly Disagree 2 Disagree 3 Neither Disagree nor Agree 4 Agree 5 Strongly Agree	
c. I make it mandatory for him or her to receive the treatment.	1 Strongly Disagree 2 Disagree 3 Neither Disagree nor Agree 4 Agree 5 Strongly Agree	
d. The patient's spouse or partner encourages him or her to get the treatment (if applicable).	1 Strongly Disagree 2 Disagree 3 Neither Disagree nor Agree 4 Agree 5 Strongly Agree	
e. The patient wants to get the treatment.	1 Strongly Disagree 2 Disagree 3 Neither Disagree nor Agree 4 Agree 5 Strongly Agree	

Survey Item	Response Options	Source/Reference
f. The patient believes that the treatment works (it helps to reduce their symptoms).	1 Strongly Disagree 2 Disagree 3 Neither Disagree nor Agree 4 Agree 5 Strongly Agree	
g. I believe the treatment works.	1 Strongly Disagree 2 Disagree 3 Neither Disagree nor Agree 4 Agree 5 Strongly Agree	
h. The treatment worked while the patient was at the NICoE so the patient expects it will continue to work now.	1 Strongly Disagree 2 Disagree 3 Neither Disagree nor Agree 4 Agree 5 Strongly Agree	
i. Other (please explain):	Free text	
There are also many things that can pose barriers to patients getting the care NICoE recommends. Please rate the extent to which you agree or disagree that the following make it more difficult for your patients to get the treatment or services NICoE recommends.		Britt et al., 2008 Schell and Marshall, 2008.
a. The patient doesn't trust TBI or psychological health professionals.	1 Strongly Disagree 2 Disagree 3 Neither Disagree nor Agree 4 Agree 5 Strongly Agree	
b. The patient doesn't know where to get help.	1 Strongly Disagree 2 Disagree 3 Neither Disagree nor Agree 4 Agree 5 Strongly Agree	
c. The patient doesn't have adequate transportation.	1 Strongly Disagree 2 Disagree 3 Neither Disagree nor Agree 4 Agree 5 Strongly Agree	
d. It is difficult for the patient to schedule an appointment.	1 Strongly Disagree 2 Disagree 3 Neither Disagree nor Agree 4 Agree 5 Strongly Agree	
e. The patient would have difficulty getting time off work for treatment.	1 Strongly Disagree 2 Disagree 3 Neither Disagree nor Agree 4 Agree 5 Strongly Agree	
f. TBI or psychological health care costs the patient too much money.	1 Strongly Disagree 2 Disagree 3 Neither Disagree nor Agree 4 Agree 5 Strongly Agree	

Survey Item	Response Options	Source/Reference
g. The patient would find it embarrassing.	1 Strongly Disagree 2 Disagree 3 Neither Disagree nor Agree 4 Agree 5 Strongly Agree	
h. It would harm the patient's career.	1 Strongly Disagree 2 Disagree 3 Neither Disagree nor Agree 4 Agree 5 Strongly Agree	
i. Members of the patient's unit might have less confidence in him or her.	1 Strongly Disagree 2 Disagree 3 Neither Disagree nor Agree 4 Agree 5 Strongly Agree	
j. The patient's unit leadership might treat him or her differently.	1 Strongly Disagree 2 Disagree 3 Neither Disagree nor Agree 4 Agree 5 Strongly Agree	
k. The patient's leaders would blame him or her for the problem.	1 Strongly Disagree 2 Disagree 3 Neither Disagree nor Agree 4 Agree 5 Strongly Agree	
l. The patient would be seen as weak.	1 Strongly Disagree 2 Disagree 3 Neither Disagree nor Agree 4 Agree 5 Strongly Agree	
m. The patient believes TBI or psychological health care doesn't work.	1 Strongly Disagree 2 Disagree 3 Neither Disagree nor Agree 4 Agree 5 Strongly Agree	
n. Other (please indicate): _____	1 Strongly Disagree 2 Disagree 3 Neither Disagree nor Agree 4 Agree 5 Strongly Agree	
Please indicate the degree to which you disagree or agree that the following would help to improve the NICoE referral process and recommendations for care.		N/A
To improve the NICoE referral process:		
a. Use electronic referral	1 Strongly Disagree 2 Disagree 3 Neither Disagree nor Agree 4 Agree 5 Strongly Agree	

Survey Item	Response Options	Source/Reference
b. Provide a link to the referral in AHLTA	1 Strongly Disagree 2 Disagree 3 Neither Disagree nor Agree 4 Agree 5 Strongly Agree	
c. Include a description of NICoE eligibility criteria on the referral form	1 Strongly Disagree 2 Disagree 3 Neither Disagree nor Agree 4 Agree 5 Strongly Agree	
d. Shorten the referral processing time	1 Strongly Disagree 2 Disagree 3 Neither Disagree nor Agree 4 Agree 5 Strongly Agree	
e. Other: _____	1 Strongly Disagree 2 Disagree 3 Neither Disagree nor Agree 4 Agree 5 Strongly Agree	
To improve NICoE's recommendations at discharge:		
a. Improve NICoE's knowledge of the availability of specific types of services at the patient's home station	1 Strongly Disagree 2 Disagree 3 Neither Disagree nor Agree 4 Agree 5 Strongly Agree	
b. Increase communication between providers at the NICoE and the home station before the patient is discharged from the NICoE	1 Strongly Disagree 2 Disagree 3 Neither Disagree nor Agree 4 Agree 5 Strongly Agree	
c. Provide home station providers with more advanced notice when NICoE decides to extend a patient's stay	1 Strongly Disagree 2 Disagree 3 Neither Disagree nor Agree 4 Agree 5 Strongly Agree	
d. Shorten the length of the discharge summary	1 Strongly Disagree 2 Disagree 3 Neither Disagree nor Agree 4 Agree 5 Strongly Agree	
Other:_____	1 Strongly Disagree 2 Disagree 3 Neither Disagree nor Agree 4 Agree 5 Strongly Agree	

Patient Survey

Survey Item	Response Options	Source/Reference
Have you ever been a patient at the National Intrepid Center of Excellence (NICoE) in Bethesda, MD, right outside Washington, DC?	0 No 1 Yes	N/A
Has a doctor or health care provider ever told you that you have a Traumatic Brain Injury (TBI) or concussion?	0 No 1 Yes	N/A
Are you currently on active duty or planning to return to active duty?	0 No 1 Yes	N/A
[IF not active duty or planning to return to active duty]: Were you medically separated (i.e., med boarded out)?	0 No 1 Yes	N/A
[IF currently active duty]: Are you currently in the process of medically separating (i.e., med boarding out)?	0 No 1 Yes	N/A
Are you...	1 Male 2 Female	N/A
How old are you?	Write in [0–99] [0–99]	N/A
Are you of Hispanic or Latino origin or descent?	0 No 1 Yes	N/A
What is your race? (*Please select one or more*)	1 White 2 Black or African American 3 Asian 4 Native Hawaiian or Other Pacific Islander 5 American Indian or Alaskan Native 6 NONE OF THESE (please describe): _____	N/A
What is the highest level of education you have achieved?	1 High school diploma or GED 2 Some college 3 Associate's degree 4 Bachelor's degree 5 Graduate degree (Master's, PhD, MD, JD, etc.) 6 Other (please describe): _____	N/A
Of which service are/were you a member?	1 Air Force 2 Army 3 Coast Guard 4 Marine Corps 5 Navy	N/A
Are/were you...	1 Active Duty 2 Reserve 3 Guard	N/A

Survey Item	Response Options	Source/Reference
[IF Active Duty]: Are you currently in a Warrior Transition Unit/Wounded Warrior Battalion?	0 No 1 Yes	N/A
What is/was your rank/rate/pay grade?	E1–E9, WO1/WO–CW5/CWO5, O1–O10	N/A
How many deployments have you completed in support of OIF, OEF, OND, or another contingency?	0–99	N/A
Throughout this survey we will ask about the care you have received for Traumatic Brain Injury (TBI) or concussion. We will use the acronym TBI to refer to head injuries. **The first few questions ask you to think back to the period of time before you went to the NICoE.**		N/A
Thinking back to how well you were feeling before you went to the NICoE, how much were your TBI and/or psychological health symptoms impacting your relationships with other people (friends, spouse, children)?	0 Not at all 1 Minimal impact 2 Moderate impact 3 Severe impact 4 Extreme impact	
How much were your symptoms impacting your work or your ability to work?	0 Not at all 1 Minimal impact 2 Moderate impact 3 Severe impact 4 Extreme impact	
When you learned you would be going to the NICoE, what was the **most** important problem you hoped to address? (*Check one*).	1 Sensory problems (e.g., poor hearing, sensitivity to light) 2 Pain (e.g., headaches, back pain, joint/muscle pain) 3 Psychological or emotional concerns (e.g., posttraumatic stress, depression, anger) 4 Concentration or memory problems 5 Speech and language issues 6 Sleep problems 7 Relationship problems 8 Other (please indicate): _____	
How much distress did [MOST IMPORTANT PROBLEM] cause you **before you started at the NICoE?**	0 None 1 Minimal distress 2 Moderate distress 3 Severe distress 4 Extreme distress	

Survey Item	Response Options	Source/Reference
The next set of questions ask about your satisfaction with the care you received at your home station before you went to the NICoE. For each statement, please indicate whether you were not at all satisfied, slightly satisfied, moderately satisfied, very satisfied, or completely satisfied.		N/A
Overall satisfaction with the care you have received for TBI and/or psychological health at your home station **before** you went to the NICoE	1 Not at all satisfied 2 Slightly satisfied 3 Moderately satisfied 4 Very satisfied 5 Completely satisfied	
The care you received before you went to the NICoE specifically to address [MOST IMPORTANT PROBLEM]	1 Not at all satisfied 2 Slightly satisfied 3 Moderately satisfied 4 Very satisfied 5 Completely satisfied	
Your relationship with your home station providers (before you went to the NICoE)	1 Not at all satisfied 2 Slightly satisfied 3 Moderately satisfied 4 Very satisfied 5 Completely satisfied	
Your home station providers' knowledge of TBI and/or psychological health conditions	1 Not at all satisfied 2 Slightly satisfied 3 Moderately satisfied 4 Very satisfied 5 Completely satisfied	
The next set of questions ask about your satisfaction with the care you received at the NICoE. For each statement, please indicate whether you were not at all satisfied, slightly satisfied, moderately satisfied, very satisfied, or completely satisfied.		N/A
Overall satisfaction with the care you received for TBI and/or psychological health while you were at the NICoE	1 Not at all satisfied 2 Slightly satisfied 3 Moderately satisfied 4 Very satisfied 5 Completely satisfied	
The care you received at the NICoE specifically to address [MOST IMPORTANT PROBLEM]	1 Not at all satisfied 2 Slightly satisfied 3 Moderately satisfied 4 Very satisfied 5 Completely satisfied	
Your relationship with your NICoE providers	1 Not at all satisfied 2 Slightly satisfied 3 Moderately satisfied 4 Very satisfied 5 Completely satisfied	
Your NICoE providers' knowledge of TBI and/or psychological health conditions	1 Not at all satisfied 2 Slightly satisfied 3 Moderately satisfied 4 Very satisfied 5 Completely satisfied	

Survey Item	Response Options	Source/Reference
What did the NICoE recommend you do to continue addressing [MOST IMPORTANT PROBLEM] once you were discharged? (check all that apply) (Note: If you have it, use your NICoE discharge summary to help you remember)	1 Talk to a psychologist or therapist 2 Talk to a doctor or nurse in a behavioral health clinic 3 See a specialist for head-related care (e.g., neurologist or TBI clinic) 4 See a specialist for pain (e.g., muscle pain, joint pain, back pain) 5 See a specialist for tests and assessments 6 See a primary care provider (e.g., your regular doctor) regularly 7 Engage in alternative therapies (e.g., acupuncture, meditation, yoga) 8 Engage in self-care (e.g., eat healthy, exercise, smoking cessation) 9 Engage in memory strengthening tasks (e.g., writing things down, keeping a schedule) 10 See a physical therapist regularly 11 See a speech/language therapist regularly 12 See an occupational therapist regularly 13 Other (please explain): _____ _____ _____ 14 Nothing was recommended 15 Don't know	N/A
[IF Nothing recommended]: Why wasn't anything recommended to address [MOST IMPORTANT PROBLEM] after you were discharged from the NICoE? (check all that apply)	1 I don't know 2 It wasn't a problem anymore 3 They didn't know it was a problem 4 The treatment for this problem is not available at my home station 5 Other (please explain): _____	
The next set of questions address the care that you have received since you returned from the NICoE.		
Thinking about when you left the NICoE and returned to your home station, please indicate the extent to which you agree with the following statements about getting the care that NICoE recommended for [MOST IMPORTANT PROBLEM].		Britt et al., 2008 Schell and Marshall, 2008.
a. The recommended treatment is easily accessible in my area.	1 Strongly Disagree 2 Disagree 3 Neither Disagree nor Agree 4 Agree 5 Strongly Agree	

Survey Item	Response Options	Source/Reference
b. My commander or supervisor supports me getting the recommended treatment.	1 Strongly Disagree 2 Disagree 3 Neither Disagree nor Agree 4 Agree 5 Strongly Agree	
c. My doctor makes it mandatory for me to receive the recommended treatment.	1 Strongly Disagree 2 Disagree 3 Neither Disagree nor Agree 4 Agree 5 Strongly Agree	
d. My spouse or partner encourages me to get the recommended treatment (if applicable).	1 Strongly Disagree 2 Disagree 3 Neither Disagree nor Agree 4 Agree 5 Strongly Agree	
e. I want to get the recommended treatment.	1 Strongly Disagree 2 Disagree 3 Neither Disagree nor Agree 4 Agree 5 Strongly Agree	
f. I believe that the recommended treatment works (it helps to reduce my symptoms).	1 Strongly Disagree 2 Disagree 3 Neither Disagree nor Agree 4 Agree 5 Strongly Agree	
g. My providers believe that the recommended treatment works.	1 Strongly Disagree 2 Disagree 3 Neither Disagree nor Agree 4 Agree 5 Strongly Agree	
h. The recommended treatment worked while I was at the NICoE so I expect it will continue to work now.	1 Strongly Disagree 2 Disagree 3 Neither Disagree nor Agree 4 Agree 5 Strongly Agree	
i. Other (please indicate): _____	1 Strongly Disagree 2 Disagree 3 Neither Disagree nor Agree 4 Agree 5 Strongly Agree	

Survey Item	Response Options	Source/Reference
There are many reasons why someone might not get a recommended treatment. Please indicate the extent to which the following have been challenges for you in getting the treatment recommended by the NICoE to address [MOST IMPORTANT CONCERN].		Britt et al., 2008. Schell and Marshall, 2008.
a. I don't trust TBI or psychological health professionals.	1 Strongly Disagree 2 Disagree 3 Neither Disagree nor Agree 4 Agree 5 Strongly Agree	
b. I don't know where to get help.	1 Strongly Disagree 2 Disagree 3 Neither Disagree nor Agree 4 Agree 5 Strongly Agree	
c. I don't have adequate transportation.	1 Strongly Disagree 2 Disagree 3 Neither Disagree nor Agree 4 Agree 5 Strongly Agree	
d. It is difficult to schedule an appointment.	1 Strongly Disagree 2 Disagree 3 Neither Disagree nor Agree 4 Agree 5 Strongly Agree	
e. There would be difficulty getting time off work for treatment.	1 Strongly Disagree 2 Disagree 3 Neither Disagree nor Agree 4 Agree 5 Strongly Agree	
f. TBI or psychological health care costs too much money.	1 Strongly Disagree 2 Disagree 3 Neither Disagree nor Agree 4 Agree 5 Strongly Agree	
g. It would be embarrassing.	1 Strongly Disagree 2 Disagree 3 Neither Disagree nor Agree 4 Agree 5 Strongly Agree	
h. It would harm my career.	1 Strongly Disagree 2 Disagree 3 Neither Disagree nor Agree 4 Agree 5 Strongly Agree	
i. Members of my unit might have less confidence in me.	1 Strongly Disagree 2 Disagree 3 Neither Disagree nor Agree 4 Agree 5 Strongly Agree	

Survey Item	Response Options	Source/Reference
j. My unit leadership might treat me differently.	1 Strongly Disagree 2 Disagree 3 Neither Disagree nor Agree 4 Agree 5 Strongly Agree	
k. My leaders would blame me for the problem.	1 Strongly Disagree 2 Disagree 3 Neither Disagree nor Agree 4 Agree 5 Strongly Agree	
l. I would be seen as weak.	1 Strongly Disagree 2 Disagree 3 Neither Disagree nor Agree 4 Agree 5 Strongly Agree	
m. TBI or psychological health care doesn't work.	1 Strongly Disagree 2 Disagree 3 Neither Disagree nor Agree 4 Agree 5 Strongly Agree	
n. Other (please indicate): _____	1 Strongly Disagree 2 Disagree 3 Neither Disagree nor Agree 4 Agree 5 Strongly Agree	
How much distress does [MOST IMPORTANT CONCERN] cause you **now**?	0 None 1 Minimal distress 2 Moderate distress 3 Severe distress 4 Extreme distress	
Please rate your agreement with the following two statements:		N/A
I have the skills, support and resources I need to improve my [MOST IMPORTANT CONCERN].	1 Strongly disagree 2 Disagree 3 Neither disagree nor agree 4 Agree 5 Strongly agree	
My trip to NICoE has positively influenced the treatment of my TBI and psychological health back at home.	1 Strongly disagree 2 Disagree 3 Neither disagree nor agree 4 Agree 5 Strongly agree	
Please rate the extent to which you would have preferred more or less of each aspect of NICoE services:		N/A
a. Length of the stay at NICoE	1 Shorter 2 3 Just right 4 5 Longer	

Survey Item	Response Options	Source/Reference
b. Number of assessments/tests	1 Fewer 2 3 Just right 4 5 More	
c. Number of individual counseling sessions	1 Fewer 2 3 Just right 4 5 More	
d. Number of group counseling sessions	1 Fewer 2 3 Just right 4 5 More	
e. Amount of computer/simulation training	1 Less 2 3 Just right 4 5 More	
f. Amount of complementary and alternative medicine (like acupuncture or yoga)	1 Less 2 3 Just right 4 5 More	
g. Amount of opportunities to build my skills to manage my TBI	1 Less 2 3 Just right 4 5 More	
h. Number of physical exams by doctors	1 Fewer 2 3 Just right 4 5 More	
i. Other (please explain): _____	1 Less 2 3 Just right 4 5 More	
Where do you currently receive the majority of care for your TBI and/or psychological health care?	1 Military Treatment Facility (MTF) 2 Veterans Health Administration (VA) facility 3 Civilian provider(s) 4 Other (please indicate): _____ _____ _____	N/A

Survey Item	Response Options	Source/Reference
What kinds of doctors or providers do you currently see for your TBI and/or psychological health care? (check all that apply)	1 Neurologist 2 Nurse practitioner (NP) or physician assistant (PA) 3 Physical therapist 4 Primary care physician 5 Psychiatrist (mental health provider who can prescribe medication) 6 Occupational therapist 7 Therapist/counselor (e.g., psychologist, social worker) 8 Speech/language therapist 9 Neuropsychologist 10 Other (please explain): _____ _____ ____ 11 I don't see any providers for these problems	CAHPS: https://cahps.ahrq.gov/Surveys-Guidance/index.html
Who do you consider your **key provider** for problems related to your TBI and/or psychological health conditions? **Your key provider is the person who knows the most about the treatment you receive for TBI and/or psychological health conditions.**	Are they a: 1 Neurologist 2 Nurse practitioner (NP) or physician assistant (PA) 3 Physical therapist 4 Primary care physician 5 Psychiatrist (mental health provider who can prescribe medication) 6 Occupational therapist 7 Therapist/counselor (e.g., psychologist, social worker) 8 Speech/language therapist 9 Neuropsychologist 10 Other (please explain): _____ _____ ____ 11 I don't see any providers for these problems	
Consider the key provider you indicated above for the following three questions:		Recommendations from *VA/DoD, 2009a*.
How often do you meet with this provider for TBI and/or psychological health care?	1 At least weekly 2 At least monthly 3 A few times a year 4 I have only met with them once 5 Never	
How long have you been seeing this provider for TBI and/or psychological health care?	1 0–6 months 2 6–12 months 3 1–3 years 4 More than 3 years	
How informed is your key provider about the care and recommendations you received from the NICoE?	1 Not at all informed 2 Slightly informed 3 Moderately informed 4 Very informed 5 Completely informed	

Survey Item	Response Options	Source/Reference
The next set of questions ask about your satisfaction with the care you have received **since you left the NICoE**. For each statement, please indicate whether you were not at all satisfied, slightly satisfied, moderately satisfied, very satisfied, or completely satisfied.		
Overall satisfaction with the care you have received for TBI and/or psychological health since leaving the NICoE.	1 Not at all satisfied 2 Slightly satisfied 3 Moderately satisfied 4 Very satisfied 5 Completely satisfied	
The care you have received since you left the NICoE specifically to address your [MOST IMPORTANT CONCERN].	1 Not at all satisfied 2 Slightly satisfied 3 Moderately satisfied 4 Very satisfied 5 Completely satisfied	
Your relationship with your current providers	1 Not at all satisfied 2 Slightly satisfied 3 Moderately satisfied 4 Very satisfied 5 Completely satisfied	
Your current providers' knowledge of TBI and/or psychological health conditions	1 Not at all satisfied 2 Slightly satisfied 3 Moderately satisfied 4 Very satisfied 5 Completely satisfied	

References

American Congress of Rehabilitation Medicine, "Definition of Mild Traumatic Head Injury," *Journal of Head Trauma Rehabilitation,* Vol. 8, No. 3, 1993, pp. 86–87.

American Psychiatric Association, *Diagnostic and Statistical Manual of Mental Disorders* (5th ed.), Arlington, Va., 2013.

APA—*See* American Psychiatric Association.

Armed Forces Health Surveillance Center, "DoD Numbers for Traumatic Brain Injury: Incidence by Armed Forces Branch," 2012. As of July 25, 2014:
http://www.defense.gov/home/features/2012/0312_tbi/chartaf_hires.jpg

Britt, T. W., T. M. Greene-Shortridge, S. Brink, Q. B. Nguyen, J. Rath, A. L. Cox, C. W. Hoge, and C. A. Castro, Perceived Stigma and Barriers to Care for Psychological Treatment: Implications for Reactions to Stressors in Different Contexts, *Journal of Social and Clinical Psychology,* Vol. 27, 2008, pp. 317–335

Carman, Kristin L., Maureen Maurer, Jill Matthews Yegian, Pamela Daedess, Jeanne McGee, Mark Evers, and Karen O. Marlo, "Evidence That Consumers Are Skeptical About Evidence-Based Health Care," *Health Affairs,* Vol. 29, No. 7, July 2010, pp. 1400–1406.

Carroll, Linda J., J. David Cassidy, Lena Holm, Jess Kraus, and Victor G. Coronado, "Methodological Issues and Research Recommendations for Mild Traumatic Brain Injury: The WHO Collaborating Centre Task Force on Mild Traumatic Brain Injury," *Journal of Rehabilitation Medicine,* Vol. 36, 2004, pp. 113–125.

Daughtridge, G. W., T. Archibald, and P. H. Conway, "Quality Improvement of Care Transitions and the Trend of Composite Hospital Care," *Journal of the American Medical Asccociation,* Vol. 311, No. 10, March 12, 2014, pp. 1013–1014.

De Groot, I. J. M., O. Even Zohar, R. Haspels, H. Van Keeken, and E. Otten, "Case Study: CAREN (Computer Assisted Rehabilitation Environment): A Novel Way to Improve Shoe Efficacy," *Prosthetics and Orthotics International,* Vol. 27, No. 2, 2003, pp. 158–162.

Defense and Veterans Brain Injury Center, "DoD Worldwide Numbers for TBI: 2012," 2012. As of July 25, 2014:
http://dvbic.dcoe.mil/sites/default/files/uploads/dod-tbi-worldwide-2012-as-of-05-Nov-2013.pdf

————, "DoD Worldwide Numbers for TBI: 2013," 2014. As of July 25, 2014:
http://dvbic.dcoe.mil/sites/default/files/uploads/2013_dod-tbi-worldwide-2000-as-of-02-26-14.pdf

DoD—*See* U.S. Department of Defense.

Eslami, M., and H. P. Tran, "Transitions of Care and Rehabilitation After Fragility Fractures," *Clinics in Geriatric Medicines,* Vol. 30, No. 2, May 2014, pp. 303–315.

Gardner, R., Q. Li, R. R. Baier, K. Butterfield, E. A. Coleman, and S. Gravenstein, "Is Implementation of the Care Transitions Intervention Associated with Cost Avoidance After Hospital Discharge?" *Journal of General Internal Medicine,* Vol. 29, No. 6, June 2014, pp. 878–884.

Helmick, Katherine, Kevin Guskiewicz, Jeffrey Barth, Robert Cantu, James P. Kelly, Eric McDonald, Stephen Flaherty, Jeff Bazarian, Joseph Bleiberg, Tony Carter, Jimmy Cooper, Angela Drake, Louis French, Gerald Grant, Martin Holland, Richard Hunt, Timothy Hurtado, Donald Jenkins, Thomas Johnson, Jan Kennedy, Robert Labutta, Mary Lopez, Michael McCrea, Harold Montgomery, Ronald Riechers, Elspeth Ritchie, Bruce Ruscio, Theresa Schneider, Karen Schwab, William Tanner, George Zitnay, and Deborah Warden, *Defense and Veterans Brain Injury Center Working Group on Acute Management of Mild Traumatic Brain Injury in Military Operational Settings: Clinical Practice Guideline and Recommendations*, Silver Spring, Md.: Defense and Veterans Brain Injury Center, 2006. As of July 25, 2014:
http://www.pdhealth.mil/downloads/clinical_practice_guideline_recommendations.pdf

Hoge, Charles W., Dennis McGurk, Jeffrey L. Thomas, Anthony L. Cox, Charles C. Engel, and Carl A. Castro, "Mild Traumatic Brain Injury in U.S. Soldiers Returning from Iraq," *New England Journal of Medicine,* Vol. 358, No. 5, 2008, pp. 453–463.

Hosek, James, Jennifer Kavanagh, and Laura L. Miller, *How Deployments Affect Service Members*, Santa Monica, Calif.: RAND Corporation, MG-432-RC, 2006. As of July 25, 2014:
http://www.rand.org/pubs/monographs/MG432.html

Hulscher, M. E. J. L., M. G. H. Laurant, and R. P. T. M. Grol, "Process Evaluation on Quality Improvement Interventions," *Quality and Safety in Health Care,* Vol. 12, No. 1, 2003, pp. 40–46.

Langlois, Jean A., and Wesley Rutland-Brown, eds., *Traumatic Brain Injury in the United States: The Future of Registries and Data Systems*, Atlanta, Ga.: National Center for Injury Prevention and Control, Centers for Disease Control and Prevention, June 2005. As of July 25, 2014:
http://www.cdc.gov/traumaticbraininjury/pdf/Future_of_Registries-a.pdf

Kaplowitz, Michael D., Timothy D. Hadlock, and Ralph Levine, "A Comparison of Web and Mail Survey Response Rates," *Public Opinion Quarterly,* Vol. 68, No. 1, 2004, pp. 94–101.

Martin, David, "Invisible Wounds," "60 Minutes," May 5, 2013, 2013. As of July 25, 2014:
http://www.cbsnews.com/videos/invisible-wounds-of-war/

McCrea, Michael, Grant L. Iverson, Thomas W. McAllister, Thomas A. Hammeke, Matthew R. Powell, William B. Barr, and James P. Kelly, "An Integrated Review of Recovery After Mild Traumatic Brain Injury (MTBI): Implications for Clinical Management," *Clinical Neuropsychologist,* Vol. 23, No. 8, 2009, pp. 1368–1390.

National Intrepid Center of Excellence, "The Interdisciplinary Model," web page, 2014a. As of July 25, 2014:
http://www.nicoe.capmed.mil/patientcare/SitePages/InterModel.aspx

———, "The NICoE Patient Welcome Guide," web page, 2014b. As of July 25, 2014:
http://www.nicoe.capmed.mil/Shared%20Documents/20130916_NICoEWelcomeGuide.pdf

———, "Refer a Patient," web page, 2014c. As of July 25, 2014:
http://www.nicoe.capmed.mil/Contact%20Us/SitePages/Referral.aspx

———, "Frequently Asked Questions About NICoE," web page, 2014d. As of July 25, 2014:
http://www.nicoe.capmed.mil/About%20Us/SitePages/Faqs.aspx

Perkonigg, Axel, Hildegard Pfister, Murray B. Stein, Michael Höfler, Rosalind Lieb, Andreas Maercker, and Hans-Ulrich Wittchen, "Longitudinal Course of Posttraumatic Stress Disorder and Posttraumatic Stress Disorder Symptoms in a Community Sample of Adolescents and Young Adults," *American Journal of Psychiatry,* Vol. 162, No. 7, 2005, pp. 1320–1327.

Public Law 110-181, National Defense Authorization Act for Fiscal Year 2008, Title XVI, Subtitle A, Sec. 1611: Comprehensive Policy on Improvements to Care, Management, and Transition of Recovering Service Members, 2008.

Riccitiello, Robina, "Casualty of War," *Newsweek,* March 13, 2010. As of July 25, 2014:
http://www.newsweek.com/casualty-war-106571

Rubicon Planning, LLC, *Army Stationing and Installation Plan*, website, undated.

Ruff, Ronald, "Two Decades of Advances in Understanding of Mild Traumatic Brain Injury," *Journal of Head Trauma Rehabilitation*, Vol. 20, No. 1, January–February, 2005, pp. 5–18.

Ryan, Gery W., Stefanie A. Stern, Lara Hilton, Joan S. Tucker, David P. Kennedy, Daniela Golinelli, and Suzanne L Wenzel, "When, Where, Why and with Whom Homeless Women Engage in Risky Sexual Behaviors: A Framework for Understanding Complex and Varied Decision-Making Processes," *Sex Roles*, Vol. 61, Nos. 7–8, 2009/10/01, 2009, pp. 536–553.

Sayer, Nina A., "Response to Commentary: The Challenges of Co-Occurrence of Post-Deployment Health Problems," 2011. As of July 25, 2014:
http://www.hsrd.research.va.gov/publications/forum/may11/may11-2.cfm

Schell, Terry L., and Grant N. Marshall, "Survey of Individuals Previously Deployed for OEF/OIF," in Terri Tanielian, Lisa H. Jaycox, Terry L. Schell, Grant N. Marshall, M. Audrey Burnam, Christine Eibner, Benjamin R. Karney, Lisa S. Meredith, Jeanne S. Ringel, and Mary E. Vaiana, eds., *Invisible Wounds of War: Summary and Recommendations for Addressing Psychological and Cognitive Injuries*, Santa Monica, Calif.: RAND Corporation, MG-720/1-CCF, 2008. As of July 25, 2014:
http://www.rand.org/pubs/monographs/MG720z1.html

Schretlen, David J., and Anne M. Shapiro, "A Quantitative Review of the Effects of Traumatic Brain Injury on Cognitive Functioning," *International Review of Psychiatry*, Vol. 15, No. 4, 2003, pp. 341–349.

Stein, Murray, and Thomas McAllister, "Exploring the Convergence of Posttraumatic Stress Disorder and Mild Traumatic Brain Injury," *American Journal of Psychiatry*, Vol. 166, No. 7, 2009, pp. 768–776.

Teasdale, Graham, Gordon Murray, Louise Parker, and Bryan J. Jennett, "Adding Up the Glasgow Coma Scale," *Acta Neurochirurgica Supplementum*, Vol. 28, No. 1, 1979, pp. 13–16.

Tomaszewski, J. J., E. Handorf, A. T. Corcoran, Y. N. Wong, R. Mehrazin, J. E. Bekelman, A. Canter, A. Kutikov, D. Y. Chen, R. G. Uzzo, and M. C. Smaldone, "Care Transitions Between Hospitals Are Associated with Treatment Delay for Patients with Muscle Invasive Bladder Cancer," *Journal of Urology*, May 14, 2014.

U.S. Department of Defense, "DoD News Briefing with Under Secretary of Defense David Chu, Lt. Gen. Stephen Speakes, and Lt. Gen. Emerson Gardner from the Pentagon," transcript, January 19, 2007. As of July 25, 2014:
http://www.defense.gov/transcripts/transcript.aspx?transcriptid=3871

U.S. Department of Veterans Affairs, *Veterans Health Initiative: Traumatic Brain Injury-Independent Study Course*, Washington D.C., 2010. As of July 25, 2014:
http://www.publichealth.va.gov/docs/vhi/traumatic-brain-injury-vhi.pdf

U.S. Department of Veterans Affairs and U.S. Department of Defense, *VA/DoD Clinical Practice Guideline for Management of Concussion/Mild Traumatic Brain Injury*, version 1.0-2009, 2009. As of July 2, 2014:
http://www.healthquality.va.gov/guidelines/Rehab/mtbi/concussion_mtbi_full_1_0.pdf

———, "VA/DoD Clinical Practice Guideline for Management of Major Depressive Disorder (MDD)," 2009b. As of July 25, 2014:
http://www.healthquality.va.gov/MDD_FULL_3c.pdf

———, "VA/DoD Clinical Practice Guideline for Management of Post-Traumatic Stress Disorder. Version 2.0," 2010. As of July 25, 2014:
http://www.healthquality.va.gov/PTSD-Full-2010c.pdf

U.S. Government Accountability Office, *Management Weaknesses at Defense Centers of Excellence for Psychological Health and Traumatic Brain Injury Require Attention*, Washington, D.C., February 2011, 2011. As of July 25, 2014:
http://www.gao.gov/new.items/d11219.pdf

VA—*See* U.S. Department of Veterans Affairs.

VA/DoD—*See* U.S. Department of Veterans Affairs and U.S. Department of Defense.

Wojcik, Barbara E., Catherine R. Stein, Karen Bagg, Rebecca J. Humphrey, and Jason Orosco, "Traumatic Brain Injury Hospitalizations of U.S. Army Soldiers Deployed to Afghanistan and Iraq," *American Journal of Preventive Medicine*, Vol. 38, No. 1, January 2010, Supplement, 2010, pp. S108–S116.